ARE YOU READY FOR GOD'S BEST?

ARE YOU READY FOR GOD'S BEST?

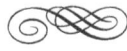

DR. CHRISTINE TOPJIAN

Christine Topjian Publishing

Contents

Some Other Titles by Dr. Christine Topjian — ix

1	Abundance Is A Mindset & It Starts With You	1
2	I've Prayed....Now What? What's Manifest?	12
3	The Holy Spirit: Our Friend, Our Confidant, Our Helper	20
4	Faith and Creating	29
5	Our Relationship with God	37
6	Being Positive	41
7	Vision and All Things Working Together For Our Benefit	56
8	Abundance	65
9	Expecting God's Best	71
10	You Are A Magnet....What Are You Calling Forth?	79
11	Strategy	84
12	Getting God's Help....Do We Need It?	100
13	"But God Isn't Around & Doesn't Know Me"	104
14	Feeling Great & Taking Care...Mentally	109
15	Feeling Great & Taking Care...Physically	115
16	Focus on Jesus	123
17	Strive for More, Better, Higher	130
18	Remember Who You Are In Christ On Those Hard Days	136
19	Congratulations, You!	149

20	Speak It!	162
21	Tech and Other Good Things	169
22	Your Ministry	179
23	The Inconvenient Moments	183
24	Don't Forget to Thank	195
25	Spend Time in the Word....On Purpose	210
26	Pay It Forward	219
27	Tithing	221
28	Christ-Based Marriages & Family Life	230

About The Author   239

Copyright © 2022 by A Success Manual by Dr. Christine Topjian

All rights reserved. No part of this book may be reproduced in any manner whatsoever without written permission except in the case of brief quotations embodied in critical articles and reviews.

First Printing, 2022

Some Other Titles by Dr. Christine Topjian

Jesus Loves You

Love & Kindness

Give It To God

Hannah Can Read e-book

It's In Transit e-book

The Chrissie Series: Chrissie Meditates & Visualizes

The Chrissie Series: Chrissie Goes Places

The Chrissie Series: Chrissie Prays

How To Be Led By The Holy Spirit

Some Other Titles by Dr. Christine Topjian

Manifest It!

I

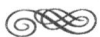

Abundance Is A Mindset & It Starts With You

I cannot overstate the importance of the abundance mindset.

Why?

Because that mindset will guide your thoughts and your actions throughout your life and if you don't have the right mindset "on" every day, you will fall short of God's best. That is, you will not have the mindset and the understanding to undertake God's best for you life and to receive His instructions for working in a decisive, strategic manner - a manner that can only come when He orders your steps.

Now, abundance does not just mean money and wealth, although those elements are part of it. In fact, abundance means feeling great, being great and doing your best every day. It means being positive and happy in mind, body, and soul. It means a closeness to God where He is there with you, helping you and guiding you. It is so important to ensure that we practice the things that will lead to those results each day because humans can sometimes naturally have a tendency to be a bit negative, and so we need to work at making sure that we are working against that.

Abundance of mind, body and soul is a collective of eating well, speaking and thinking positively, having the right relationships, fitness and spirituality. Oftentimes, when people say spirituality, some assume that we can't be referring to the Bible and to the wisdom that is provided in the Bible, but we are definitely referring to that. God is a Spirit and therefore being spiritual necessarily means being connected to God.

We were created to be whole, to be in connection with God and to be in connection with one another. This social connection, in particular, is one reason I feel social media has become so prevalent and important - because we were created for that social connection. That connection to God is also needed, which is why I believe people are often searching for that "higher power". I used the word needed in the previous sentence because need denotes something we cannot live without; we were never meant to live outside of relationship with God.

You see, God has put so much good in us. So many skills and talents in each of us. We were all created for life, happiness, abundance and goodness and He has given us the skills, talents, brains and abilities to do, to be and to have all that He has called us to. So many of the things around us, especially in nature, are positive, life-affirming things. When I feel low or like I need a little pick-me-up, I sometimes go for a walk in nature and I am very mindful and grateful for the pure and clean oxygen the trees provide, the flowers, the animals, the grass, the air, the sky and so much more. These things are so very important to each one of us because they remind us of nature and of goodness, and they provide an outlet for breath, for fresh air and for pure oxygen, tenets of good mental health and wellness. This is also why yoga touts and encourages the breath so much - because in breath, we are inhaling life and hope and freedom and goodness right into our mental health and into our being.

So, friend and reader, abundance is a mindset, it's a connection to

God. It's mind, body, spirit and soul, and ultimately, it's our amazing access to God who is a Triune Spirit consisting of God the Father, Jesus the Son and the Holy Spirit (Who lives inside of us when we are baptized).

Take time to feed your soul the abundance that can only come from God. Take time to walk in nature, to talk to God, to eat well and healthy, to do your fitness workouts, to engage in meaningful, life-affirming relationship and friendships, and above all, don't forget that our #1 connection is with God, the Provider and Source of all that is so good!

The abundance mindset begins with you and is all about your relationship with God. You see, God has already provided everything: health, wealth, financial prosperity, family, friends, good opportunity, good breaks, and more. He provided all of these things in anticipation that you will be needing them and wanting them. They have all been provided to you in the spirit realm. He has also provided us with the opportunity for relationship with Himself and all we have to do is tap into this relationship (activate it, if you will) and you will see His gifts, guidance and abilities come to be in your life!

We were meant to rely on Him and to do life in tandem with Him. In John 15:5, the Bible says **"I am the vine; you are the branches. If you remain in me and I in you, you will bear much fruit; apart from me you can do nothing."** This does not mean that God is mean and wants to withhold good things from you. Quite the contrary. It means that He wants you to rely on Him and His ways and His goodness in doing things so that when opposition comes (and it will - we all know life can be full of challenges), you are ready to respond and you have the power of God in your corner to defeat the opposition and to make your way over to success and accomplishment.

To provide you with an example, I knew that the Lord was guiding me to executive produce my own media production. I knew that this was His will because I had been feeling it quite strongly and throughout my Doctoral studies, I knew that this was an important part of the journey. When I called in to the organization where I needed to register this production, I met with some pretty fierce opposition. Now, this was an organization that *I was already part of*, so this opposition really shouldn't have been happening. But it was. I had unfortunately come across a woman who answered the phone and said some terrible things, essentially wanting to shut the phone in my face. I tried to explain without being rude that all I wanted to do was exercise my rights to create this production and that I knew there was nothing in the rule book that said I couldn't. This lady wasn't having it. Instead of hang up in frustration, I prayed in my mind, asking the Lord to open this door, if it was His will. Not five minutes later, this lady apologized to me for her rudeness, and began answering my questions on how to complete the form in the right way and to send it in right away.

You see, opposition did come and it was fierce - but it was no match for what God could do and did do!

You have opposition in your life too. We all do...we all have things we want to accomplish but we are having difficulty and experiencing challenges because that's what happens here in life. You have to rise above it and you have to call on the power of God to help you because that's what He has guided us to do.

Now, there are a few things you need to do in order to call forth and claim all that He has for you. You need to:

- **Pray for it**
- **Stay in faith that you will receive it**
- **Speak the words of victory with your mouth**
- **Wait and watch for it to manifest**

I will now explain each:

- **Pray for it**

    When we pray for something, we are engaging God into conversation and we are asking about what we are supposed to do. We are filling Him into an active conversation. Prayer, after all, is a two-way conversation - we have to communicate (via our thoughts or words) and then we have to listen to what He is saying, prompting us to and guiding us to.
- **Stay in faith that you will receive it**

    When we stay in faith that we will receive something, we wait expectantly for it. We listen for it. We take actions that are going to lead us to achieving our goal. This is part of the faith that God is waiting to see us demonstrate. When you stay in faith that you will receive it, what you are basically saying is "God, I know You are guiding me to this and I am going to take all the actions You guide me to to getting it." When we do this, God gets a little smile on His face because He can see that we are stepping out in faith.

- **Speak the words of victory with your mouth**

    Our words are very powerful. We can call amazing things into being. Scripture tells us that "life or death is in the tongue" (Proverbs 18:21) and so we can call forth life (positivity) or death (negativity) with our words. When you speak positive, life-affirming words, imagine and rightfully assume that you are getting steps and steps closer to the realization of your goals.

Speaking words of victory with your mouth and thanking God for what He is doing that you cannot see are all part of the strategies required to move forward to the accomplishment of all He has called you to do.

I remember when I was helping a family member through a difficult time, I tried as much as possible to remind them that this is just a tough part and that the reward for persevering will be great. I encouraged them to remember that every time the going got tough or things seemed difficult. In the end, everything would be just fine and they would enjoy the good feelings of knowing that they persevered through something so difficult.

- **Wait and watch for it to manifest**

When we stay in faith and we do the things that we are called to do, we are then supposed to wait (sometimes it's a brief wait and sometimes it's a little longer) and we will watch it come to be in our lives. In this area (and I hope you all learn from a mistake I made in the past), I want to tell you that the manifestation of what you are waiting for in faith may not look exactly (or anything like) what you think it will look like. Things often tend to look different and for that reason, we sometimes miss out on our blessings.

A friend of mine wanted to be married a great deal and was actively looking and dating. She ended up meeting a wonderful man and after a brief courtship, she announced to me one night that she was getting married. As a close friend of hers, I was invited to the wedding and it was simply a beautiful evening. After their honeymoon, things were still good between them but I started to notice her looking a little more sullen and sad. When I asked her during one of our outings what was going on, she announced that she and her husband were separating. I was shocked. At this point, I already had a strong relationship with the Lord and I was dumbfounded because I knew that these two were meant to be together. They also hadn't been married long and she was willing to throw in the proverbial towel without much of a reason, without having had any counseling, without much of anything. I tried to talk things out with her, tried to reason with her and encourage her to go to marital counseling, talk things out with him, etc., but she was not open to any of it.

What am I saying? The manifestation of her dream happened but it took a little bit of work (as all marriages do) and so it looked different than she had thought it would and so she decided to walk away.

Walking Away Can Be Hard

Many people will say that sticking with something is a challenge but I have news for you: walking away is sometimes even more challenging. When we walk away, we are saying that there is no chance this thing can ever be retrieved and I'm done trying to retrieve it. When we walk away, we are saying that we have already relied on God and that there is nothing that can be done to help. That is true only in the most rare of cases.

This concept of sticking with it can be applied in every life case we deal with, from relationships to money and everything in between. Taking the example of a marriage (again) for a moment, we are called not only to love each other, but also to cherish each other, to listen to each other, to pray for each other, to keep no record of wrongs, to support each other (even when it is inconvenient) and much more. A fantastic book by author Gary Thomas called Cherish, outlines this concept beautifully and the book teaches us why and how to cherish our spouses for the most solid kind of marriage we can ever hope to have. We were never supposed to do marriage with just you and your spouse - it is effectively a union between you, your spouse and Jesus. Why? Because Jesus is there in Spirit to help you both have patience, understanding, to help you both when you or your spouse stumbles, and more.

Another example is dealing with money and finances. We are all called to tithe and to provide offerings of 10%. Some may argue that this is an Old Testament concept and that it is not in use today. Please try it out and see the effects of what giving provides in your life. See the good that the money you give does and see if God will not in turn bless you.

Take the example of your job or your career. You may be getting frustrated that the promotion is taking so much longer than you could fathom or that you are being held back or that you are doing everything you can to show how dedicated an employee you are but that lucky break hasn't happened yet. You may be tempted to walk away. You may be called to walk away but why don't take that question to God first and see what He speaks into your soul? He will be able to tell you if walking away is the right thing to do or if you should stick with it and you will be able to get a sense of it.

A lady I knew had been getting increasingly frustrated that the promotion she thought she was supposed to be getting wasn't coming. She began to complain to me that she had been waiting for the promotion for years and that she felt that God was leading her to stay where she was and to not get discouraged. When I tried to minister to her and to talk her through this, she had said that she had been waiting for over six years for the promotion. I sensed that something was off. When I probed a little, she explained that she had begun at the company five and a half years prior. I reminded her that not many people get a promotion after being with a company for six months. When we started talking through things, she also admitted that she had been less-than-professional toward her boss on a few occasions and I needed to gently remind her that people who talk to their bosses that way may not be able to expect a promotion anytime soon. As we took a step back and looked at things from a more holistic, global and realistic view, she began to see how little actions and steps she could take would lead to better performance reviews and ultimately, to that promotion that she wanted.

What am I saying? When you are thinking of walking away from something, check-in with God to see what He is saying about your situation. Ask Him and let Him show you what the reality of the situation is or situations are, before you do anything. We may not be seeing everything as it needs to be seen and we may be requiring some added perspective on things that can only be achieved when we go to the greatest Mind in the world.

How To Have the Strength

Everyone goes through hard and challenging times and needs God's strength to get through it. So, how do we (faulty humans as we are) have the strength to endure? We rely on Christ.

Some of what Christ provides:
* strength
* peace
* love
* a more global understanding of your specific situation
* a reminder of who you are in Him
* insight
* understanding
* comfort
* wisdom
* a way
* the bigger picture of what others are dealing with
* an opportunity to repent for your own wrong-doings

When we rely on Christ, through the Holy Spirit, we are fortunate enough to have THE highest power in the world in our corner helping us, fighting our battles, helping us to have the strength to endure all that we need to. That is why when we are getting married (the greatest union as instituted by God) we present ourselves at the altar of God and we are asking the Pastor to unite us into union with this person and with God, *because He is and will always be in the union with us*, helping us through all the difficulties we will ever experience. We were never supposed to handle the union with our spouses as just the two of us.

So, when you are embarking on this union called marriage or any endeavor, the point is that no matter what stage you are at, you are called (we are all called) to have this union with Jesus at the center, operating in us through the Holy Spirit.

How so? Let me illustrate.

Let's say today you have an argument or a misunderstanding with your spouse and you leave the home feeling angry or not heard or misunderstood. We sometimes won't understand why our spouse is acting the way they are and we sometimes need strength to understand, to be patient, to gain perspective and more. It is God who gives us that understanding, patience, perspective and more. It is He who gives us all that we will need for our marriages to be healthy and successful not just on your wedding day but far into the future.

A lady I was ministering to regularly ate earlier in the evening without waiting for her husband to come home. She would be eating away, finishing her meal and would set aside his meal for him. She didn't ask him if this bothered him in any way or if he would prefer that she wait for him for dinner and maybe have a healthy snack while she is waiting. I encouraged her to pray about this and to seek the Holy Spirit to see if maybe she should have been waiting for her husband to have dinner with him. She complied and prayed about it. She had a talk with her husband about it, asking him openly if he didn't like that she ate without him on a regular basis and he said that he felt relieved that she asked about this because yes, in fact, he really would prefer to have dinner with his wife when he came home and would really have appreciated if she had a small snack and waited to eat her full dinner with him. She was very surprised that he felt that way and so because of her love for him, she decided she would wait for him so that they could eat dinner together.

We may not even realize things that may be or are on the minds and hearts of our spouses but it is so important to make sure that we pray for wisdom from the Holy Spirit and that we check-in with our spouses, even on those things that we think are obvious and that we may take for granted.

Taking the example of the lady who wanted the promotion, she needed to check-in with God and use His wisdom to gain a better understanding of the situation, so that she could navigate the situation carefully and thoughtfully. We are not supposed to rely on our own understanding.

What does this have to do with a book about the prosperity mindset or abundance? Plenty! If you want to have abundance and prosperity, you are highly encouraged to include Jesus and the Holy Spirit into every part of your life, because we all need that help and support.

The following Scripture helps to remind us of the invitation to rely on Christ and that His personality is both gentle and humble:

28 "Come to me, all you who are weary and burdened, and I will give you rest. 29 Take my yoke upon you and learn from me, for I am gentle and humble in heart, and you will find rest for your souls. 30 For my yoke is easy and my burden is light." (Matthew 11:28-30)

2

I've Prayed....Now What? What's Manifest?

What does to manifest mean? In the context of Christ, it means to bring something to reality that which already exists in the Heavenly realm. It means to be able to see the evidence of it in the physical sense, in tangible form. You see, according to Scripture, every good thing has been given to us. When Jesus died on the cross at Calvary, every good thing was already given to us so we are not asking God to give this to us - it has already been provided. That changes how you should be praying. You are not praying to receive these things. You already have them. You are just calling them forth into being present in the physical sense (this is the manifesting step).

That's why I say that the abundance mindset starts with you because it is your mindset and your way of thinking and believing that tells you that everything you need is available to you and that God has already done the work of providing. Now that it is provided, you need to see it (manifest it) in real life. In other words, *assume it is already yours because it is.* Speak like it is done. Walk like it is done. Move like it is done. Think like it is done.

When you pray for something that is in God's will, know that it exists in the Heavenly realm, and that it's only a matter of time before you see it in the physical realm. And yes, there are actions you need to take in the physical realm in order to see that thing (or those things) manifest in the physical realm. For instance, the Bible clearly tells us that you need to work in order to get financial abundance, (Proverbs 10:4) **"Lazy hands make for poverty, but diligent hands bring wealth."** This means that you have to go out and work if you are able - whether it's working for a company, working as an entrepreneur and having your own business, whatever it is. You have to work for the Lord to bless the work and pay your tithes as well. (Proverbs 12:24) **"Diligent hands will rule, but laziness ends in forced labor."**

I was speaking to an actor friend of mine who said that he felt fortunate because he works five days a week most weeks while some others don't, or struggle to find work. I asked him what he does differently to work five days per week at a craft that he loves. He said that he hustles and he goes looking for work, he doesn't just wait for it to come to him. He calls, emails and texts his acting agents on the regular, making sure that his name is at the top of their minds and that they know that he is available for work. This man has made the decision that acting is his calling from God and as such, he knows that idle hands and no work will get him nowhere. Instead, he hustles, he networks, he strives and he works very hard to make sure that he is booked for roles he is right for. He is constantly messaging with the decision-makers in the field to make sure that he is seen, he communicates his availability, he communicates that he is prepared for the role, and he works. As a result, God has richly blessed the works of his hands, as he told me that he makes a very healthy living out of his acting work. Good for him!

Continuing for a moment on the subject of the works of your hands being blessed. Everyone is called to do something great, and great can be in any field: politics, education, dance, engineering and science, math, languages, and the list goes on and on and on. You know or you may have an idea of the skills you have inside of you and for each one of those skills, it's a wonderful blessing to know that you have the ability to make a living from that work, for the benefit of you and those around you.

For instance, you could be a great chef - you have been given the great gift of creating some of the most delicious and innovative dishes in the world and your calling could be to use it to be a great cook in a restaurant, while another person is a gifted dentist and can do wonders for the dental needs of all those that are fortunate enough to be in his or her dental chair. Alternatively, you can be a great chef and your calling is to do short order cooking while another chef's calling is to develop a great new pastry and market that as a frozen food or another option is to be a chef in a busy, upscale restaurant in some part of the world. We do not all have the same calling or the same paths because we were not all created with the exact same gifts (and that's great because we all have specific talents and skills that we can bring forward). Another way to put it is that we each have our own calling and we are totally unique in that - you may very well be the only person in the world who can bring that particular gift to the world and to make the world a better place with your particular calling and gift(s).

The trick is to decipher, through your relationship with Jesus and with the Holy Spirit, where your particular gifts lie and to see how God wants you to utilize those gifts.

God wants to communicate where your gifts are to you - He's not trying to keep that a secret, so you would be wise and do well to ask Him about them and to let Him reveal them to you in His own special way or ways. He can communicate it to you by putting that fire inside of you, by bringing you the opportunity, by bringing you someone who encourages you to do that very thing, by opening the doors to schooling that trains you in the skills you will need to have, etc.

I also want to point out that you may very well have more than one gift. Many people have a number of wonderful and awesome gifts and so they are meant to do more than one thing. I knew of a man who spent the first 40 years of his career being a general contractor and then realized that he also had the gifts of making people laugh, so he decided to spend his next set of years as a comedian on stage. So, what I'm saying, friend, is that you need to ask God where your gifts lie and how you should utilize those gifts to honor God. He will also be the One to open all the right doors you need to make something happen.

I'll take the example here of a friend of mine who felt the calling to be a police officer. Her family was not enthusiastic about the idea for the same common reason many other family members wouldn't: she would be putting her life on the line each and every single day. Her loved ones wouldn't know whether she would be coming home alive at the end of each day. Still, she felt the call very strongly and she knew that this was where she needed to be. Among the other challenges she was facing, she also shared with me that she didn't have the money to pay for the schooling or training required, so she was at a loss. She decided to "**be still and know that He is God**" (Psalm 46:10) and slowly but surely, one by one, the pieces began coming together and not only did the funds come together for her to pay for the training, but her family met some of the family members of those who were on the force and began to discover ways to become more comfortable with the idea of her new career. Fast forward a few years later and she is now a general sergeant on the force and she is as in love with her job as possible.

More Than One

I want to make it clear here that we can each certainly have more than one calling. A person can be a gifted doctor, comedienne, talented chef, teacher, mother, caregiver, lawyer and more and there is nothing wrong with doing all of these things at the same, or at different times, depending on how God is leading you. He will guide you as to how and when and where He wants you to do each of these things and in ways that will honor Him. I was at a comedy club one night and enjoying the comedic stylings of a brilliant comedian. While he was in the middle of his set, someone from the audience called out "that's my former Math teacher". The comedian blushed a little while on the stage and then shared with the crowd that he was also a teacher, a volunteer firefighter and wore a few other hats. I found this inspirational and amazing that this man wore so many hats and was serving all the different parts of his personality and fulfilling the areas of his life where he felt called.

I used to be very surprised when God revealed to me that He had more than one calling for me. I think it stems from the fact that I watched my parents do one profession for all of their professional lives and so I assumed that if you are doing one thing, that that would be all you are or will be doing for the rest of your professional life. Not so.

If God has brought you more than one calling, great. Embrace it. Love it. He has given you the skills to do more than one thing and that is a blessing. A lady I know used to always think that being a mother and a stay-at-home wife was her calling in life and as she was doing it, she used to tell me just how happy and how grateful she was to be doing it every single day. Until one day, circumstances changed and her very sweet husband let her know gently that a little more money was needed for the family finances. He respected the fact that she loved being a stay-at-home mom and told her that if that's what she wanted to keep doing full-time and only that, that that would be fine but that they would need to make some adjustments. I advised her to pray about it and she did, asking the Lord to reveal things to her through me. God said very clearly that she could easily do part time work creating greeting cards and memorabilia (she had a knack for doing that) and that she could set up a little home-based business. I told her about this and she accepted that but she wasn't sure how to get started. I advised her to start with step one and take it one day at a time, and not to worry about seeing the whole proverbial staircase.

She went shopping for wholesale supplies and I watched as little by little, the old tricks for creating stunning greeting cards that her grandmother had taught her as a child flooded back to her and she began to make those greeting cards with the supplies she had just bought. She began working on this business in her off-hours, when the kids were at school, when other chores were done and on weekends when her parents or her in-laws took the kids out for a few hours. She began creating the most stunning greeting cards of very good quality, hired a person to help build her business a website through which she could sell her cards and memorabilia items and with simple social media strategies, she began to get the word out about her products. The orders started coming in and she was so thrilled. She was having a great time making these, felt like she was honoring her grandmother with the skill as well as honoring the gifts that the Lord had put inside of her, and felt relieved and happy that she was starting to contribute to the family income with the revenues. She mentioned to me that she had never expected to make money with this skill that she had learned as a child but that this push from God was what she needed to get started with this wonderful endeavor.

In sum, God will open the way to make things happen for you and to bring things together in a way that you wouldn't be able to. He is the God who opens doors for us, allowing us to do His will. We have to do what we can here on earth and then let Him take over and do what we cannot do.

> We have to do what we can, and then let Him do what we cannot.

Our Expectations

I have come to realize that our expectations also have a big role to play when it comes to how and when we think we will see something manifest. I experienced this myself when I thought something was going to take much longer to appear and so I wasn't paying enough attention or being very mindful about it so when it did appear, I let it slip through my fingers. When people say "God's timing" we may immediately get the idea that God's timing means way later and not for now. It may mean that but one of the problems with this line of thinking is that when we think that something won't be happening soon, we tend to not pay much attention to it (as I did). Not paying much attention to it usually then means that we aren't thinking much about it and so that thinking can cause us to straight-up miss it when it does appear. The unfortunate thing about this is that when you miss the opportunity, it may not come around again too quickly, and so we are then faced with the unfortunate situation where we will need to wait again for it and this time, keep our eyes peeled.

The fact is: you receive in the same measure as you expect. If you expect something to take 5 years to happen, it will. If you expect it to take 1 week to happen, it likely will.

If you are thinking to yourself *"Christine, I don't believe I will ever meet the right person. It's too hard, dating sucks, she's just not out there or he's just not out there."* Well, you have already lost half the battle. She is out there or he is out there and you do need to ask God how you will meet this person, when and what He wants you to know about this. Now, that may mean dating but it may not. I know plenty of people who didn't even really date their God-directed person but did end up with the one that God intended for them without dating because the circumstances called for it to be so. To illustrate, a friend of mine's parents met, had their first date and got married all within 6 months and they have been happily married for over 40 years.

It doesn't always happen in the same way for everyone and so realistically, just because everyone else is going about doing it one way, it doesn't necessarily mean that it's the right way. *"How do I know what the right way for me is?"* Ask God and then let the Holy Spirit speak to your heart. For more information about this, please feel free to reach me via my website at DrChristineTopjian.com. I have helped a number of people understand God's will for them because it is one of my gifts from the Lord.

3

The Holy Spirit: Our Friend, Our Confidant, Our Helper

The Holy Spirit is there to be our Friend, our Confidant, our Helper and our Guide through every step. God has placed the live Holy Spirit in us so that we have our Guide and we can know what to do with confidence at every step. Now, you don't have to see the entire staircase in order to take the first step.

This particular visual has proven to be very helpful to me and to many I have ministered to:

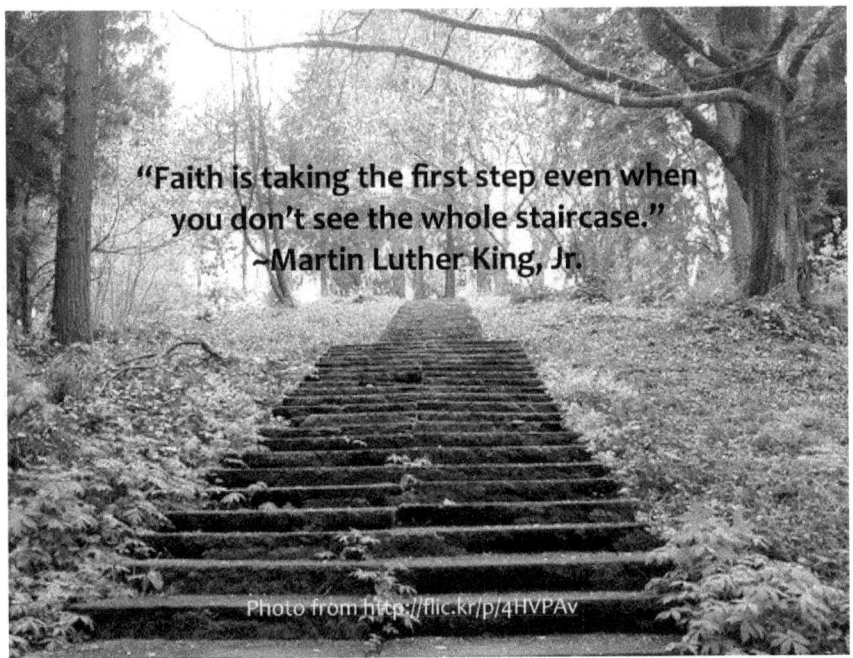

"Faith is taking the first step even when you don't see the whole staircase."
~Martin Luther King, Jr.

Simply put, it means that there is a full staircase which is representative of our entire path. Because of all the steps, it means that there are many things we will need to do in order to make it to our goal and to experience what each step of the staircase holds. This holds true for all types of goals because for everything, there is a process. Taking each step without being aware of what the next one will hold is a matter of faith. We don't know what will be there but we have to have faith and we have to ask the Holy Spirit to guide each of our steps. The Holy Spirit will show you each and every step to take, when to take it and how to take it. He is our Guide. Because we do not know what is waiting for us next, we are relying on the character of God to help us and to guide us and we are relying on the good character of God. This is what we call "blind faith".

I also know that through our close relationship with Christ and with the promptings of the Holy Spirit, we are guided to do all the right things - but if we don't actually do them, if we don't actually take the actions and do what God tells us to do in the time frame and in the way that He is guiding, we will be missing out on God's best and on His provision for our ideal lives. **These are such important concepts because really, they tell us how much God loves us, how He wants the best for us and how we can be standing in our own way.**

The best example of this that I have is from a friend of mine. He had a friend with whom he was completely in love with. I received a vision one afternoon that he was, in fact, meant to be married to her. She was the love of his life - she just hadn't clued into it yet and he wasn't yet close enough to God to understand that this was in fact, God's will for both of their lives. I had received clear guidance that I was to go to his workplace (he worked on his own and he made his own schedule) and to tell him about this, gently. I was tasked with guiding him to a relationship with the Holy Spirit and to begin taking that first proverbial step.

I did this. It was not easy.

We had a deep conversation in his office at work and he did admit to me that he was, in fact, secretly in love with her. I was dumbfounded that I hadn't seen it earlier but hindsight is 20/20 and the revelations of the Holy Spirit are also perfect. She was a woman of faith and he didn't know much about faith but I remember my words to him: start your own faith journey, talk to God and begin reading the Bible in anticipation for when she realizes things and she comes around. I said to him: "You don't have to see the whole staircase…just take the first steps."

He did. He took the first steps and he began to pray, to read the Bible and he began his faith journey. I am happy to report that just a few months later, his best friend did realize that she was in love with him and today, they are happily married with children.

What am I saying?

Do like this man and take the first steps….they will lead to the best for you because that is God's will for you: the best.

So, going forward, we all need to be vigilant and to keep our eyes open to the promptings of the Holy Spirit because the manifestation and fulfillment of our prayer can happen at any time and if you miss it, you may have to go back to the drawing board and start over.

> In fact, everything in life in Christ is just like that - we are manifesting at the rate that we believe we should be.

The Holy Spirit Guiding

A friend of mine was trying to get into a teacher's college. He believed that he would have to wait months and months in order to get even a word acknowledging his application. I suggested to him through the promptings of the Holy Spirit that it doesn't have to take that long and in fact, he can even select a school that has rolling admission. He followed up on the suggestion and sure enough, not 2 months later, he began teacher's college. Today, he has been teaching for over 14 years. You see, had he believed that it was so hard, that it would take months to hear back, that there was no other way it could happen than the way he saw, and not having listened to the promptings I advised him of through the Holy Spirit, he would have held himself back from trying, from hoping, from applying. Instead, he listened and followed up on the suggestion and found himself in school barely two months later.

Another girl I knew was looking to get pregnant with her first. She wanted a baby really badly but found out that she and her husband were dealing with some infertility issues that she hadn't previously known about. She felt like she was never going to get pregnant. Month after month, she got her period, and when Mother's Day rolled around, her reaction to a lack of a baby was heartbreaking. She was having a really hard time coping. I told her the same thing I'm telling you today: expect it, speak as though you have it and watch it manifest itself. I told her that I would one day soon be helping her with her baby, and that she was going to really enjoy being a mom. She also asked the Pastor of her Church for her input and the Pastor prayed with both she and her husband so that they could have a baby, however way God intended them to. Sure enough, about 6 months later, the surrogate she had selected announced that she was pregnant and 9 months later, they had happy and healthy twins!

Sari was a young woman who was aching for love. She wanted it badly and she always told me about how she believed in true love and in soulmates. I told her that I agreed with her about true love and soulmates and I knew, from my own faith and prayers, that God was leading her to a specific man. I gently began guiding Sari to the possibility of this man and that it may be worth her time to give this man another look, since he was already in her life. She was not hearing it. She wanted no part of it. Instead, she decided to go online and to begin trying to meet men through a dating app. I knew in all of my being that she was wasting time, that the man for her was the one I had guided her to because of the promptings of the Holy Spirit but she didn't want to accept that. I again reminded her to see things differently, to look at how well this man had treated her over the years and that even though he wasn't exactly what she thought her future husband looked like, that he was ultimately the right man for her. Today, Sari is single and continues to scour dating sites aimlessly.

Stay in faith….pray for it, pay attention to the promptings of the Holy Spirit to see what you need to do to make it happen….. and let it manifest....don't get in your own way! You may not see a way but God has a way.

One more example I will provide is another woman I was helping with finding the love of her life had family members suggest she go online to find her husband. Because of my close relationship with God and the promptings of the Holy Spirit, I knew that that was not the right way for her. I suggested a different avenue and that she look a little closer at a particular man who was in her church group with her. She was in total disbelief about his potential to be "the one" for her because he was younger than her and she had never thought of a younger man as a romantic potential. I urged her to look again and reminded her about how he had been there for her during a very trying time in her life and how she had been extremely grateful for this man's help during that trying time. She did ultimately decide to open herself up to a possible future with him. Fast forward about 2 years later and she let me know that she had realized that God was consistently guiding her to the same man, the same one I had advised her to look at more closely. Today, they are married and they are proud parents of not one but two happy and healthy babies.

Working On It A Bit Each Day

In order to see the results we are looking for, we need to take consistent, Holy Spirit-inspired actions. The fulfillment of our dreams will not come from sporadic, inconsistent actions here and there. A painter needs to paint regularly in order to become a great painter, a writer needs to practice their craft a little each day and a surgeon does not become the best by doing one or two surgeries. Instead, we need to take action a little bit each day, working toward excellence in whatever field we are in and working toward identifying what we are doing well, and where we need to improve.

As such, God provides for us each and every day, via words of wisdom, visions, inspiration, motivation, opportunities and much more. When we ask Him to show us the actions and steps that are needed each day, He gives us a list of things we need to do daily in order to achieve what we need to achieve. Checking in with Him each day allows us to receive His guidance each day and to know that we are on His schedule to accomplish things.

So, when you are waking up and about to begin your day, here is a suggested prayer to ask the Lord to guide your steps for that day:

> Lord, what would You have me do today? What needs to get done, in what order, when and how, so that I am accomplishing all that I need to? Please guide me on what needs to be done when so that I am doing all that I need to do.

Pray this simple prayer and you will sense and feel the nudgings, if not full directions and instructions. Write down the promptings and what you get as a response. As part of my Doctoral studies, I had to get into the habit of doing this each morning, after my quiet and special time with Jesus. I had to write out the day's work and I had to make sure I was doing each thing the way He guided, when He guided and how He guided. It was tremendously important to me to ensure that I was doing each thing on the list because God is very time-specific and will only guide you to do something when the time is ripe. If you don't do it within the time window provided, you will be missing out on His best.

You see, God is a God of order: things need to be done in a certain organized sequence. He always has a good reason for step 1 being that step and the other steps following. So, find out what your step 1 is and move on that step. I suggest you write down each detail that He gives you because you will need that as a task list that you can simply check-off as you go! Write it on your tablet, smartphone, journal, a piece of paper, whatever. Write it and do it.

Ask Many Questions

Something else very important that I learned through my Doctoral program is to ask many probing questions. God will tell you if you ask Him. If you don't ask, there is a high chance He won't tell you and you will see later how not having had that piece of information has put you at a real disadvantage.

So, ask all the questions, ask how something has to be done, ask when and where and why something has to be done. The Holy Spirit will respond and will guide you.

These are just some of the Scriptural names of the Holy Spirit and in which Scriptural book these references can be found:

1. Breath Of The Almighty (Job 33:4)
2. Counselor & Comforter (John 14:16,26; 15:26)
3. Spirit of Counsel (Isaiah 11:2)
4. Eternal Spirit (Hebrews 9:14)
5. Free Spirit (Psalm 51:12)
6. God (Acts 5:3-4)
7. Good Spirit (Nehemiah 9:20; Psalm 143:10)
8. Lord (2 Corinthians 3:16-17)
9. Power of the Highest (Luke 1:35)
10. Spirit of Christ (Romans 8:9, 1 Peter 1:11)
11. Spirit of Glory (1 Peter 4:14)
12. Spirit of Yahweh (Isaiah 11:2, Isaiah 61:1)
13. Spirit of Grace (Zechariah 12:10, Hebrews 10:29)
14. Spirit of Knowledge (Isaiah 11:2)
15. Spirit of Truth (John 14:17, 15:26)
16. Spirit of Life (Romans 8:2)
17. Spirit of Understanding (Isaiah 11:2)

As we can see, the Holy Spirit has many functions and many roles in our lives. When we see and acknowledge all that He provides, we realize how great a gift it is that God has provided this Spirit for us.

It is also important to check-in and to see if you have done everything as it needs to be done. If you are anything like me, I can certainly miss some details along the way and I learned to ask more deeply probing questions and to get more information!

4

Faith and Creating

Ask yourself what you are creating with your words and your thoughts each day.

Faith and creating are synonymous with each other. In other words, when we have faith, we are literally creating - or I should say co-creating, with God. When we imagine something, we begin co-creating it. When we speak something, we begin co-creating it. That's why so many books tell us to keep our thoughts and our words positive because if we spend time thinking about negative things or we speak negative words, we are literally creating negative in our lives. We are inviting negative into our lives. So, as much as possible, keep your thoughts and your words positive. Even when you begin to say negative things or have negative thoughts, catch yourself and consider changing your thoughts and your words into positive ones. Here are some examples of speaking positively over yourself, and your day:

Negative: I'll never learn this. What's the point...I'll never make it.
Change to: I am a work in progress and each day, each hour, I am getting better and better. It may take me some time but I will get it.

Negative: I won't ever move up in this company. I am always going to stay where I am.

Change to: I am working on learning so that I get better and I can be considered for a promotion with this company. I am excited and working hard.

Negative: I failed another test. I'm no good. I'm stupid.
Change to: I will make a study plan and do a little each day. Maybe I can consider getting a tutor or a peer tutor or even asking someone I know to help explain this. I will get this and I commend myself for not giving up. I am smart and I will not give up.

Negative: Everyone around me is moving on in life and I am stuck.
Change to: I am happy for those around me and my time is coming too. I believe that the good things God has for me are chasing me down. I am praying for God to show the steps I need to take to get the things that are meant for me.

Negative: My marriage is never going to get better. What's the point?!
Change to: We are working on communicating and we are seeking some counseling to be better communicators, to be more honest with one another and to working hard to make this a cherish-filled, Christ-centered marriage.

Negative: The medical report is terrible and I don't see any progress.
Change to: The medical report doesn't have the final say; God does and He can heal me even if the report says that things are dire.

Negative: I'm going to fail this test.
Change to: I'm going to dedicate myself to studying for this test and then when I get my results, I'm going to review any errors I made to get better and to understand where I went wrong in order to prepare for the next test.

Negative: I'm worthless.

Change to: I am made in the likeness of God and He loves me so very much. Jesus thought and thinks I was and am to die for. I am a masterpiece.

Negative: I am never going to get married....it's hopeless.
Change to: I am going to pray for God's will for me in terms of marriage and I'm going to follow all that He says to meet and be with my soulmate. My God-given spouse of my dreams is out there and is waiting to marry me.

Negative: Everything is terrible and isn't going to get better.
Change to: Things may be challenging now but I am going to pray to Jesus and let the Holy Spirit guide me on how I need to handle everything and do as the Holy Spirit guides. I am going to dedicate myself to doing what the Lord says because He loves me and wants the best for me.

Friend, the words and the thoughts we think are vital to the quality of life we wish to have. There is a lot of negativity out in the world and there are many challenges to overcome, no matter what your dreams or goals are, but that's why we have the gifts of the Holy Spirit and of Jesus and we can rely on both to get us through. We have to develop resilience in order to overcome these things.

I know that it can be difficult to keep your words and your thoughts positive when you're going through difficulties but that's also where your self-discipline and instilling reminders for yourself can be very beneficial and handy. Your attitude about something is so important and we can either see the proverbial glass half empty or half full. For instance, if you choose to see things positively and you can see that you are moving in the right direction, you can be glad about that. In the words of Mrs. Joyce Meyer, "You may not be where you need to be but thank God you're not where you used to be."

Each step forward is just that...a step forward and each thing you choose to see positively and as an opportunity will be so.

Why, God, Why?!?!?

In a recent conversation with a friend, we got into a discussion where she alleged that God was not fair and that she had to stop believing in Him. I explained to her that it is important to pray and to try to understand why things are happening the way that they are. I also tried to gently and respectfully remind her that we don't always turn to God for what we need before we need it, so when things don't go our way, we cannot then put the blame on Him for what has transpired.

This is such an important point to emphasize: **God believes in each of us and loves each of us more than we can possibly understand. He sent His only Son, Jesus, to die for us because He loves us so much.** So when we say that we don't believe in God because the world is so broken or He allowed this to happen or that to happen, we have to look for a moment (just a little bit) at our own actions. Have we ever really turned to Him? Have we ever really let Him into our hearts and asked Him to talk to us? If we have, have we fully and completely obeyed what He has guided us to?

We each have free will and when we never choose to go to Him with our problems, to ask for advice, to ask for wisdom and more, we may be taking on the stance that we know better. I mean this as respectfully as possible: we don't know better. We have human minds and we can only see so far. God is All-Knowing, All-Seeing and is Omniscient and Omnipresent - which means that He knows all and can see all (including the future).

To illustrate with an example, an elderly couple had a dream to start their own business. They wanted to open a cafe and sell pastries, coffee, etc. The wife had gotten years of compliments from family and friends on her pastries and now they wanted to turn this gift of hers into a bona-fide business. When they prayed about it, God led them to open up shop at a location that was near their house and let them know that this was the ideal and perfect location for the cafe. They weren't sure exactly why He was guiding them to this location because even though it was close to their home, the location was quite big and was more expensive than they were looking to spend. The communication was clear, though: this was His ideal location for them. So, with blind faith, they set up shop where He guided.

Business was very good and was running smoothly but the couple still didn't understand why this was the ideal place for them. The rent seemed quite high to them and there was much more space than they thought they needed. Then, covid happened.

Because of the additional space and the way the layout of the store was, they were able to re-open much sooner than other cafes because the added space allowed for more social distancing. During the time when they were only allowed to do deliveries, their business remained extremely steady due to the neighborhood patrons continually ordering from them, and because of their location, they got the government tax breaks that helped them do well instead of just staying afloat. The couple would not have been able to make ends meet with the other location they were thinking to open that was smaller simply because the context and allowable opening restrictions during covid would have been completely different in the other location and would not have allowed for the benefits they were enjoying in the larger location.

Their human minds could not have seen what was to come, but God did. That's trust and that's God's wisdom at work and because they obeyed, their business is thriving today and they are doing exceptionally well.

Why You Aren't Seeing It Yet In the Physical

If you are not yet seeing it in the physical realm, please check to make sure that you are not getting in your own way. Ask yourself the following questions:

1. Do you believe it has already been accomplished in the God-given sense?
2. Are you spending time with God to see what He is saying to you about this?
3. Are you doing all the things you know you're supposed to be doing?
4. Are you doing all the things in the time frame that He is guiding you to do?
5. Are you thanking Him ahead of time and giving gratitude for having provided the solutions?

If you are doing all the right things you are guided to do, take heart and know that your blessing is on its way.

Don't Just Follow Others

One of the most important things I want to emphasize in this context is respectfully, please don't think you automatically know the answer to what is needed. For instance, many believe that in order to be the best doctor, you have to go to this school or to that one. Or that to find your soulmate in this day and age, you have to go online and begin online dating. But did God tell you to do that? What if you ask Him and He tells you to do something completely different because He has another way for you? If you don't check-in with the wisest mind, you will surely miss out on His best and His way for you.

This happened to a lady that I was ministering to. I will call her Naya. Naya was very motivated to find her husband and because she knew that I have a relationship with God, I asked God on her behalf. Naya was very excited to know the answer. The answer came and I knew exactly to whom she was being guided to. I told her and her response: great! She was already crazy about him so she was happy to hear that he was the right one. In fact, even though she had been a self-proclaimed atheist, she had known without a shadow of a doubt that this man was the one for her and that her chance meeting with him could only have been orchestrated by God because she knew that there was no other possible explanation for how things happened and how events and timings lined up for her having met him. I felt we were moving along very well in the endeavor to get her married to this man. As time passed, she would speak to me about his ways, his words and more. She was deeply in love with him and I seemed to understand the way this man was operating pretty well, so I was able to help her dissect what he was saying and what it meant.

I remember she said to me at one point "*Christine, this is a lot of work!*" and I told her that while I agree that it was proving to be a lot of work because she also had to pray for him, that she needed to continue with it and stay the course. I advised her of how even though this man was the right person for her, that he did need some work (which is not at all an abnormal thing) and that many prayers were going to be needed to transform this man into the man of God that he would need to be in order to be ready for a loving, committed, monogamous and Christ-centered relationship with her. I advised her that he needed many prayers and that this would take time. She stayed the course for a few months and then, despite seeing some solid changes in him as a result of much prayer, she decided that she did not want to stay the course. She decided that she did not want to continue doing the work that was eventually going to lead to them being married and having a solid marriage. Today, Naya is single and has shared with me that she will eventually be going online to find herself a spouse who wouldn't require the work that this man does, even though she knew in her heart that she would never love another the way she loved this one.

5

Our Relationship with God

Our relationship with God is the most important relationship we will ever have. He created us, He sustains us, and He knows and loves everything about us, even those things that we may find hard to love about ourselves.

God is always waiting there, looking to have that close relationship with you. He wants to help you and to be part of your life every single day. If you don't give Him and yourself that opportunity, you are literally missing out on the most important relationship of your life.

God Speaks To People Today And Every Day - Are You Listening?

Joyce Meyer of Joyce Meyer Ministries said it perfectly: *"God is talking but who is listening? He is the Source, the One who created you, He is the be all and end all. Are you listening to what He has to say in your life or do you think you know better?"*

I was talking to a family member of mine who was refuting what I was saying on a really important topic but I knew I had heard God correctly because I had prayed and asked the same question several times and over an extended period of time for confirmation and for assuredness. Finally, I asked my family member *"Who knows better, you or God?"*

To my surprise, it actually took him about 4-5 minutes to answer that question and was almost debating about knowing better than God. I asked him to reflect on that and to think twice about claiming to know better than God. I think that people who don't know God might assume that He wouldn't be interested in the "small" details of our lives but this is simply not true - God is interested and wants to be invited into literally every single part of our lives because He loves us so much and only and always wants the best for us.

DETAILS!

One of the things I learned the hard way is that God is very detailed and loves to be asked questions. When we don't ask questions and probe further, we are missing a lot of information because God doesn't always just supply the answer - He waits for us to ask and to probe and to seek more detail and information. I learned early on in my walk with Him that we need to probe deeply, thoroughly and consistently and to ask lots of questions and then follow-up questions so that we can get the full picture of what He is guiding us to.

"Are we puppets?"

Going back to the conversation with my family member, I remember he asked me this question when I spoke of God knowing better. Are we puppets? Of course not. We all have free will and we are certainly not puppets. God did give us a brain and a mind, as well as the ability to reason and to have free will but if I am making the argument that God knows better and He's guiding you to this and not that, then don't you think you need to listen?

Unfortunately, we humans sometimes think we know better than God. I can say that because I have, in the past, thought (arrogantly) that I knew better or that God was wrong or somehow misunderstood the situation. When He was dealing with me about staying away from a particular man He had told me very clearly was meant for someone else, I pretended not to hear it, prayed that He would change His or his mind, and much more. Let me tell you that what I got was totally slammed. I got slammed because God had warned me that I was on the wrong track with this man and when He warns you to stay away from something, it really is best to listen because He is trying to save you from heartache and from unnecessary disappointments.

> **I have realized that when you ask God but then go your own way, you will get slammed and it will hurt! The hurt and the pain will last. Take it from me: don't go your own way!**

The Scripture says **"Lean not on your own understanding but by every word that comes from the mouth of God."** (Proverbs 3:5-6)

You see, God has a wonderful plan for each of us. He knows the ways we should go and when we don't go that way, it's like we are veering off-course. We are going the wrong way. As many of you know, when we go off the wrong way, it is a painful experience and we do end up having to take time and effort to correct our course, to change and to shift gears, and to get back on the right track. Further, the effects of going the wrong way can and sometimes do last for years, because we have already set a certain course of action into motion and this would be very hard to correct. So, the best thing to do would be to ensure that we are following His promptings and doing things the best way possible based on how He guides us to doing them.

Document What You Have Already Done

One thing in particular that I find really important is to write down what I've been guided to do and what I have done already. I actually use a checklist system in order to write down the steps that are needed and that I was guided to, and I check off one by one the actions I undertook to complete what was already done towards those ends. I also write down the date on which I was guided to take the actions and when I actually took the actions because this helps me to stay accountable to myself that I am doing everything I need to do for the attainment and fulfillment of my goals. It's amazing to look back and see where you started, the steps that you have taken so far, and to see how much further you have to go but bearing in mind that you've already come this far and to motivate yourself to keep going. It's also really important because it helps you understand and contextualize all the steps that you needed to take in order to get where you need to be.

I will sometimes also write out how I felt when I was undertaking particular actions. When I know that an action has been particularly thrilling for me, I will write that down because I want to take note of how I felt when I did that. It is a way of congratulating myself for a job well done. This also works when you take a difficult action and once you've taken it, you can now count it as done and you can now reap the benefits of that difficult time. For instance, when I do a workout that has been particularly difficult and where I really pushed my body, I look back and realize that I pushed myself and that I will reap the benefits of that and I help myself to remember to appreciate the results because I remember that it wasn't easy to get there.

Documenting helps you stay accountable, helps you stay motivated and reminds you of how far you have already come. It's also a great way to keep track of your progress and obedience to what the Holy Spirit has guided. You can use it as an example piece for others who may be struggling with their goals.

6

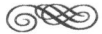

Being Positive

Having the right outlook in life is so important. There are many bad things going on every day: people dying, new diseases, killings and shootings, people acting dishonestly, people stealing from one another, death and division, etc. It's easy to think about those things and to get down and depressed. It's easy to remember the negative and to dwell on those things, especially when things are not going the greatest. But what we need to do is to tune into the channel where we remember good things and where we anticipate and expect good things to happen to us. It's too easy to dwell on the negative: *"My house payments are due"* or *"I have bills to pay." "My kids are off-course"* or *"How am I ever going to pass this exam?"* Yes, we all have troubles in our everyday lives and things that worry us but if we dwell on the bad instead of focusing our attention on the good, on what we have already accomplished, on what we have already managed to achieve in the past, then each thing will feel like an insurmountable task.

So, **change the channel and keep positive**. Keep the positive memories at the forefront of your mind, ready to replace the not-so-great memories whenever you need. Remember the happy days you spent with your friends and family, the good breaks you've received in life, the meaningful conversations, the laughter of a child, the day something unexpectedly wonderful happened in your life, how you accomplished something, how you managed to deal with something successfully, and so much more.

I knew of a woman who was extremely down about herself and her family. She was always so negative, so sure that something else bad was going to happen to her, another tragedy to befall her. I kept impressing upon her (for years, in fact) to be more positive, to believe in God's promises for happy days, for goodness and not for evil, for prosperity in all senses of the word. I reminded her that the words she speaks today will help her become the person she is tomorrow. Unfortunately, she did not heed my reminders and to this day, she has a very negative outlook and again unfortunately, all the negative things she spoke over her life have all come to pass. Every last one of them. She lost her house, refuses to work (even though she is very capable of working), her child got off-course and stayed off-course, today he has no future and has been kicked out of school with no plans to return, and she has decided to fold her arms and not take any action that will change the course of her life for the better.

It's Not Too Late

If you identify with the description just above, know that it is never too late to change the channel. There could be a million things wrong and you still, each day, you have an opportunity to change the channel and to do better, to be positive, and to speak and say positive words over your life.

It Takes Time to Get Out of the Slump

If you are in a slump, it will take time to get out of it because you have likely spoken negatively and thought negatively for some time. But it isn't something you can't get out of, nor something that needs to stay status-quo. Again, all you have to do is change your words and your thoughts. I also want to point out here that you don't initially have to believe everything you say when you are speaking positively over yourself, not believe every good thought when you think it, but begin. It will take time for the tide to turn but **the sooner you begin, the sooner the tide will turn**.

Another woman I knew felt that she didn't have much going for her - she didn't come from money, she was bright but not at the top of her class or anything, and she said she had average skills but was never truly amazing at anything she set her hand to. But what she did have going for her is that she was incredibly positive and worked so hard. She worked so hard and she stayed so positive that she overcame all the challenges that were in front of her. She worked hard at school and graduated one of the top of her class. She put in so much positivity into all she did and she ended up marrying a wonderful, kind and successful man who was attracted to her positive demeanor, and she always did her best to pay it forward and to be good to others. By speaking positively over her life in a consistent manner and following the promptings of the Holy Spirit, she got into a top college, worked very hard and lived her dream of being a tremendous nurse, author and poet and she is buying her first home even before the deadline she had set for herself. She once told me how much she relied on Scriptural promises and on God's goodness for His promises for a good future and not to harm her.

The Scripture is very clear:

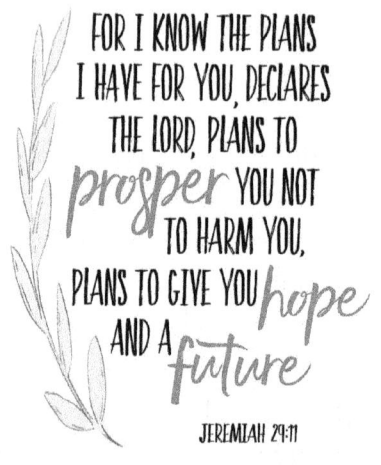

This means that God wants to prosper us and give us a future. That means that we were and are meant to have a good life by the One who created us. Will it always be easy to get ahead in life? Certainly not, but what we do have is a promise from our Creator that He will work to give us good things if we only use the tools He has put in front of us.

Negative Thoughts Will Come

One of the most frequent complaints I hear from people is that negative thoughts come and that's why I want to really tackle this issue just a little more before moving on. Everyone gets negative thoughts but it's what we do with those negative thoughts that makes the difference. Do we accept them or do we discard them and focus on what is good and on moving forward to better? That's the main difference. **If we focus on what is good (and good will mean different things for different people), then we will definitely feel better and have a more bright, positive outlook.** When we choose to dwell on the negative (yes, this is a choice), we will get more and more down. We will have more and more days where we feel down, depressed, etc.

Change the channel and focus on what is good. This is an exercise I decided to try one night. I started getting negative thoughts and feeling down, so one thing I chose to do is to turn off my phone, close my eyes and focus on what is good and positive. I chose to do a short meditation where I brought to mind all the good things in my life, my accomplishments, my amazing relationship with God, the good I already had in my life and much more. I chose to tune everything else out and to focus on the good. Within a few minutes, I began to feel better. I began to focus on each of the positive things that my life and my faith offered me in that moment:

- Relatively healthy
- Enjoying my time on my walk in nature
- Asking God to help me stay positive
- Being grateful for my relationship with Jesus
- Being sensitive to the promptings and guidance of the Holy Spirit
- My family
- My friends
- The fact that I am, in a few months, going to be a first time auntie
- The money I do have and being able to pay my bills as best as I can
- My loving cat
- Much more

You see, friend, I could have stayed dwelling on the negative, on the bad thoughts that did come and will inevitably come again. But I chose to purposefully change the channel and think about the positive things instead.

An Exercise for You

Take a few minutes right now and think about the positive things in your life now. They can be big or small, it doesn't matter and when you're done with your list, I suggest three things:

#1: Keep the list handy so you can turn to it when you feel down.

2: Allow yourself more space to write more things because that list is going to grow.

#3: Include absolutely everything (even being able to take a deep breath of fresh air)

#4: Keep several copies here and there if you would like.

Write out the things that make you happy:

Because images and visuals are important and one of the ways God speaks to us, I'd like to give you a few images that are meant to be merry-making and happy thoughts-provoking. If you can, take a moment to write down the positive emotions and thoughts that come to you with each. Remember, this is an exercise designed to remind you of the good things in life, and if these things are not yet in your life, perhaps they are things you would like to bring into your life, write that down as a future goal. If the image evokes unhappy feelings, feel free to skip it or work to change the meaning of the image to make it more positive for you.

You will see a suggested interpretation that is from me about why I decided to include these images and a suggested interpretation of the image. You can use my interpretation as your own or you can choose your own.

Image 1

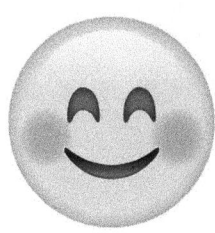

Suggested interpretation: In Christ, we are never invited to "figure it out ourselves". In fact, we are advised to never worry but to trust all in the Lord. So, I decided to put this in to remind you to not worry but to leave your problems in God's hands after you take the actions He guides you to take. Also remember that after you give the problem to God, you are invited to take it easy and to enjoy your life (hence, the happy face).

Image 2

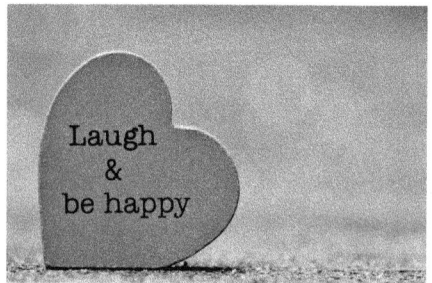

Suggested interpretation: Laughter is so very important to feel good and it's such a healthy thing to do for our mind and mental health and well-being. Being happy is also a conscious choice that we can work on being as frequently as possible.

Even when people have been diagnosed with major illnesses, they are invited to surround themselves with happy-making things and with things that promote laughter as one means to heal themselves, whether that is to watch a comedy show, a funny movie, to laugh with your friends and family, read a comic or book of satire, etc.

Image 3

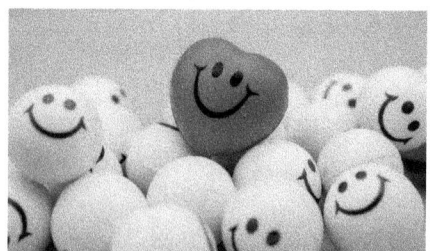

Suggested interpretation: Having at least one day where you can put on a happy face would be powerful. Smiling is an energy and it is contagious, so imagine how much good you can do for yourself and for others (even total strangers) by just providing them with a happy face or a smile as you go by.

You can also select a day with your loved ones that you can call "Happy Face Day" and you can all make an effort to smile at each other, and at others as you each move through your respective days. Even if people don't tell you that you made their day better, know that it is very likely that you did!

Image 4

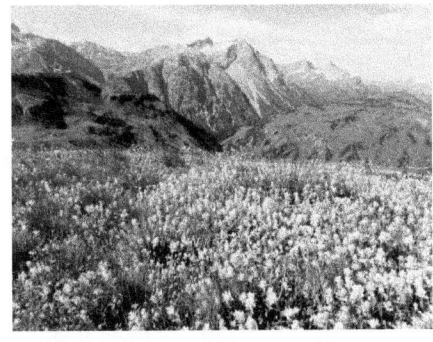

Suggested interpretation: Nature. Clean. Breath. Breathing in the natural air is so cleansing for our soul. Even just having an image like this in front of you can be such a wonderful reminder of good mental health and well-being. To some, that open road can also be a road that invites a wonderful cardio activity such as jogging and a great opportunity to bring you peace and mindfulness, helping you get distance and better perspective on anything you may be dealing with.

Seeing Visually

We are visual people. In general, people interpret and process visuals more quickly than words. God is also One Who loves to use visuals, and for this reason, He gives us visions, which are basically visual representations of what He wants to bring to earth and to us. A vision can come to you anytime and anywhere and when He gives you one, it's wise to pay attention to the details and to look and see carefully (I usually focus in on certain details as though I have a magnifying glass).

Visions are images of things (events, and happenings) that God wants to bring to earth. Let me clarify that point: He may want to bring someone's spouse or someone's new job and He may give them a vision of their wedding day or He may give them a vision of that new job, but if the person doesn't accept the vision or doesn't do the right things to help them make that vision a reality, then that person would likely miss out because of something they didn't do.

This was one of the greatest learning points I ever had to really understand because I thought that if the vision is there, it's a done deal. Wrong. You have to help it manifest. You have to act like you already have it, You have to ask God what you have to do to get it, You have to ask God to help you manifest it. Otherwise, it's something God wants to bring to come to pass, not automatically will.

This is also one of the ways we co-create with God. Co-creating means that something exists in our imagination but has not yet been released into the world yet - we are waiting for it to physically manifest in our reality and our world but by accepting and focusing on the vision He gives us, we are a couple of big steps further along to the realization of our dream. I also cover the topic of manifestation much more thoroughly in my book, Manifest It!

When God gives us a dream or a vision, He is giving it to us because it is something that He wants to bring to come to pass in our lives or something He is warning us about may happen and so if we don't want it to happen, we need to take action against it, such as praying for Him to not allow that action to take place. He gives visions because He wants us to have those moments of enjoyment in co-creating with Him. It is truly one of the greatest gifts He has given mankind because to co-create means being able to bring the great things He wants to give us to come to pass. We would be very wise to use our God-given abilities to bring good things to come to pass. These means include prayer, meditation, visualization, and gratitude.

Remember, this is also an example of receiving God's best: accepting and following the vision He gives and doing what is needed to bring about the fulfillment of those visions.

So whether it's the spouse you are looking for, or the baby you are looking to have or the program you are looking to get into or the new work opportunity you want or anything else, all of these can be included in the visions that He gives. Visions are also God's way of letting you know He wants to bring you out of something, so He is telling you what you need to do to get out of it or prevent it from coming in the first place.

"Christine, can I give myself a vision? Can I see it myself vs. waiting for God to give it to me?"

You can create your own visual but pray to make sure that you are including the information, details and particulars that He wants you to have. Why do I say that? Because you may be seeing one thing that you think is great but in the meantime, He wants to bring you something better. Remember that His ways are not our ways and His thoughts are higher and better than our own, so if we don't ask Him for details about it, we are likely missing out on His best.

Another thing you can do is to continue the vision He gave you and ask Him for more details on the vision He gave you. So, if you know or feel strongly that He gave you a vision of something He wants to bring to pass, you can easily engage in that vision more by repeating it and evoking that image in your mind again, using the same pieces and details He originally gave you.

He Did It Before

I'd like to use this opportunity right now to remind you that God has already brought you some wonderful things into your life and if He has done it before, He will do it again.

This would be a great time to think about all the good things He has brought you and challenges you overcame. You may now think of some additional things you would like to write down or add more details to the things you already have.

Some people leave out things like mobility, the ability to breath in and out, being able to live independently, being able to eat, laugh, listen, etc., but these are major and important things that we need to take inventory of and be grateful for because while you may have it, someone else may not and I think it's pretty safe to say that they would love to have it.

So, please take a moment and reflect on your list of blessings right now. You can jot them down here or take your smartphone or your journal and jot them down there. Make it personal to you and meaningful.:

My list of good things and challenges I have overcome:

If you'd like, ask Him now in prayer to show you in as much detail as possible, the things He has planned for you.

Here is a suggested prayer that you could use in order to pray to understand what He has planned for you next:

Lord Jesus, I would like to know You (better). I am asking You to come into my life and my heart and to speak to me through the Holy Spirit about what good things You have planned for my life. I want to follow You and I want Your best for my life. I am asking You to speak to me about your best and to show me (with clear step-by-step, detailed instructions) how to get there. In Jesus' name. Amen.

Write down what you see and get here in the section below. Even if it is not audible instructions but you get impressions, something like a visual, etc., write it down:

_____

_____

_____

_____

If you need additional space (which is great if you do), use additional paper or type on your device and keep the train and flow of thoughts going. This is such an amazing exercise because it should bring to the forefront of your mind and to the forefront of your thoughts the wonderful things you would like to do and that God has set on your heart.

7

Vision and All Things Working Together For Our Benefit

When we see vision or get communications, we may get emotional and that's fine. I remember when God showed me a vision of my female friend being "the one" and marrying her male best friend, I was thoroughly convinced that God had been communicating with Me for months that this is the man for her and was telling her so, through me.

This is how I got the vision: I was lying on my very comfortable couch at home when I began to see what felt like flashes of a picture coming to me. It was as if God was literally presenting me with a movie-like image and I could see it pretty clearly. The vision included them getting married, with her family and his family being so happy and joyful that both sets of parents had tears in their eyes. I could literally see the tears of joy on her family's and his family's faces. What was happening in the scenario was completely clear and evident to me. No words were needed - I knew what was happening and I remember getting emotional about it because I could see the happiness on the faces of both families and my friend and her love in their wedding attire. There was no doubt about what was happening in the image. It was amazing.

I wondered how I would come to see this part or all of this come to pass because I know God has a way of bringing these things to your attention, one way or another. I knew that He would bring me an update on things at some point and in His way. I had not spoken to her in some time but sure enough, weeks after I had gotten the vision, I was sitting and watching tv one night and a random commercial came on and the tagline in the commercial said "In this week's episode, Carla got engaged". Carla also happens to be the name of the friend in question. My body came alive and I was wondering if this was a communication of the fulfillment of the vision. I prayed about it and sure enough, received confirmation that it was. I was really surprised at how God brought me this information. I would never have expected to receive it in this way.

Real Life Confirmation

I usually like to receive real-life confirmation of the fulfillment of any vision. I did communicate with Carla after that time and she did confirm her engagement to me and that it had happened exactly on the night when I was watching that commercial. Amazing!

God Has Ways

God has ways of accomplishing things that we cannot fathom, and that we may not initially understand. He uses people, circumstances and events to change us and to transform us. He uses people to make us see things differently, to help us realize things and to remind us to keep His promises top of mind. His ways are amazing and He is never limited by the natural laws of physics (think of Jesus walking on water).

One of the things that is so amazing is when He gives us dreams. Dreams are another way that He gives us a visual of something He may want to bring to pass. If then, for example, you have a dream about something, it could very well be that that is something that is meant to happen in your life, a blessing God wants to bring to you. Dreams are also a phenomenal way God uses to cause you to pay attention to something that He is warning you away from. I remember a bad dream I had some time back about something bad happening to my brother and how it felt like a warning from God. God will often give us a warning before something bad happens for the purposes of us warning the person to make some changes or to do things differently. I knew that this was a warning that if my brother didn't pay attention to what was going on, that things were not going to go well for him in this regard. It was an opportunity for me to help him shift gears and to give him time and a heads-up to get back on the right track about an opportunity that was in front of him.

God always wants what's best for us and He will always guide us to what is best for us. He will also give you warnings when something bad is coming your way as a means of preparing you and of helping you see how He is protecting you. When you pay attention to these things, He will find ways to spare you the unnecessary from happening to you.

Your Attitude Matters....A Lot

When I received the dream warning for and about my brother, I could easily have gotten very negative (I got a bit negative but then a friend reminded me that God was giving me time to warn him to switch gears and to help him). Instead, I decided to pray about it and see what I could do to help.

Your attitude towards everything matters a lot. As one of my favorite pastors, Joel Osteen said, your attitude and whether you are going to be positive make a very big difference. I could have turned away and said *forget it* and decided to stop serving God but I didn't. I decided to rely on the awesome character of God and remain focused on what He was trying to communicate to me and what I needed to do with it. It's the same with anything else we are doing and how we choose to trust in God. Staying positive, thinking positively and speaking positively or being negative, thinking negatively and speaking negatively.

Here are some examples:

Instead of:
This will never work, what's the point in trying! **use** *I am going to work really hard and work toward this*

Instead of:
Nothing good ever happens to me **use** *I have had challenges but I know God will help me through this and I am going to pray*

Instead of:
I never get good breaks **use** *I am the recipient of all kinds of good things*

Instead of:
Every day sucks, nothing good happens **use** *Today is going to bring me a great and wonderfully happy surprise*

Instead of:
I've never done well with this, I should give up **use** *I am praying for God to help me do a great job and break this pattern*

Instead of:
I can't quit this bad habit **use** *I am working through this and asking God for His help to see myself through this*

Instead of:
My kids are off track - what's the use?! **use** *God is helping me turn this around*

Instead of:
I hate this job and I am never going to get anything better **use** *I am going*

to see how I can get better work and how God can open the doors for me to get a better position

Instead of:
I am never going to lose this weight **use** *I am going to work each day at getting fit and working out and eating well, which I know will help me lose all the weight I need to*

We all have bad days and we all have things that are not currently working well for us. Change your thoughts and stay positive. Things do take time to turn around and we definitely will need support. All of the following things are available to help us through difficult times, and this is not a completely exhaustive list:

- Access to prayer 24/7
- 24/7 access to the wisdom of the Holy Spirit
- 24/7 access to talk to God about anything and everything that is bothering us
- Access to friends and family who can not only stay positive with us but can pray with us
- Access to prayer teams who are ready and willing to pray for us and with us via different Ministries (more on this just below)
- Keep our perspective happy and expectant of the realization of that good thing
- Helpful sermons, books, devotionals and prayers to help make things easier and to help us understand
- Good, Bible-based Churches that teach about Scripture and how Scripture explains the good life we are meant to have in Christ

Prayer Ministries

Prayer Ministries are there to do just that: help us by praying for us. All you have to do is log on with an account or call in to a number that would be provided, mention the prayer you have and off it goes. Prayer Ministries work consistently at praying for the needs of all people. All you have to do is reach out in faith and they will help you by praying for your needs. I have used a variety of these services many times over the years and am always grateful that they exist. Many prayers of mine have resulted in being manifested because these people helped me.

Choosing Where To Give Your Attention

Also remember that we have the choice on which channel we choose to pay attention to. Just because the bad thoughts, the doubts, the disappointing reminders come, the frustrations linger, it doesn't mean we have to accept them or allow them to stay there. We can choose to tune in instead, to think happier thoughts, and choose to speak happier words.

According to research, people are generally more likely to remember negative thoughts and events more easily. That's why we have to work at being mindful and ensuring that we keep our focus on the good things, and that we can see things positively, even in the midst of not so great times.

I remember I was facing an almost four thousand dollar charge for a new furnace for my home. It was a lot for me and I knew I had to take care of it sooner rather than later because the cold weather was already starting to loom. I was only thinking about the money flying out of my bank account when my uncle who was visiting suggested I keep at the forefront of my mind the fact that I would have a brand new furnace in the home, I would be adding to the property value of the home, I would be helping to ensure that we didn't get any unpleasant surprises (like an old furnace breaking down in the middle of the winter) and all the other things that could happen. He also helped remind me that I am blessed to be able to have the money to make the payment in the first place, even though it would mean a considerable financial setback.

It definitely helps to have someone or people who are positive in your corner to help you see the positive side of things.

More on Seeing

When we see something for a sustained period of time, we are co-creating. Something first needs to be created in our minds before we are going to see it appear in real life. In Proverbs 28:18, Scripture says "Where there is no vision, the people perish: but he that keepeth the law, happy is he." This means that without receiving vision, people will perish because they don't have a vision of things to come. Visions give hope and hope means that we are looking for something that will come to be. Scripture is telling us that we are to have hope, in the form of vision, to see and expect things to come to pass.

A woman I know received a vision about the man she was meant to be with. Because she was a new Christian, she didn't really understand what vision was, so I took the opportunity to explain it to her. She seemed open and amenable to knowing more about visions, that she was receiving one and why she was receiving it. But when she saw that things were taking longer than expected for her to realize that vision (to actually experience it) she decided that while it was cool that she had received a vision, that she did not want to keep on track to the actions needed to fulfill the vision.

This was hard for me to watch because I had tried to minister to her many times, to explain what was going on and that she was taking the wrong way. She was going to miss out on God's best and she said that she sensed that she was doing that but that staying the course and working on getting the realization of the vision was too hard. I asked her to stay positive and I asked her to make sure that she was staying the course, that in 10-15 years from then, she would be happy she stayed with it because even though the fulfillment of the vision was going to take time, she would ultimately hugely benefit from it. To my disappointment, she decided that she did not want to stay the course.

When you are fortunate enough to receive vision, it is wise to ask God those probing questions we had talked about earlier. God is called the Teacher and we are welcome (in fact, invited to) ask the Ultimate Teacher questions. The Holy Spirit is also called the Counselor because He will counsel us as we go, whether 2 am or 2 pm.

Paying Attention to Warnings

As already mentioned, God sends us warnings to help us. He wants to see us happy and well and does want us to avoid bad things.
He sends us warnings to keep us safe and to let us know if something is not right. Ignoring these warnings is not a very wise course of action.

Allow me to illustrate: years ago, I had received a warning about staying away from a particular man because the Lord told me that he was no good for me and that I would only get hurt by him. The warning was clear and consistent in that I got it several times. I sensed and knew it was from God. It was a clear warning to be careful of something that I knew deep down was not the right thing for me.
I unfortunately, at the time, did not listen. I decided to go ahead and pursue things with him and in the process, ended up discovering some very negative and destructive things about his personality. I discovered that he lacked empathy for even the most basic things, that he was unkind in nature and sensed that he would be willing to stab anyone in the back to get himself ahead. I later found out that he did betray people to get ahead, that he did many unkind things to people I also knew and that he was exceptionally unkind to people who were trying to show him kindness and thoughtfulness. He did many things that I did not find attractive, things that did not jive with my personality in any way. After I realized that the warnings were very correct, it took

me some time to get myself out of that and to be set back on the right path again. The pain, suffering and time lost that I experienced didn't need to happen and could easily have been avoided had I been paying attention and listening to God's warnings.

8

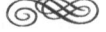

Abundance

God has always intended us to be abundant. Going back to the time of Adam and Eve, we can see how they had every abundance they could have wanted but because of disobedience, they lost a lot. Let's learn from that and practice being grateful each day. Things may not be perfect in any of our lives but we have the choice to focus on the good and to live abundantly with what we do have, and so we can always help ourselves to do better.

When I speak of abundance, I don't just mean money. Abundance is:
* good health
* good relationships
* feeling happy
* feeling fulfilled
* feeling better connected to God
* having a fulfilling career
* having a healthy family
* piece of mind
* having the time and the ability to do simple and joyful things
And much, much more

Many assume that when people speak of abundance in life, that it only or mostly focuses on money and I want to be clear that while money is part of it, I don't mean only money. If we only have money and we don't have the other things, then we are not abundant and we do not have what we need. In fact, many would argue that without health, we can have all the money in the world and it won't mean much.

How we get abundance is also important and thinking and speaking positively will definitely go a long way in helping us feel and be abundant. Take a moment right now and think about all the things that you currently have that help you feel abundant.

Write them down here. One of the greatest things about activities like this is that you can look back on your list a day, a week, a month, a year or years later and see the things that you had jotted down. It helps you see how you have evolved and how you have changed, including taking stock of the good things that you have. I also encourage you to write the date on this entry, so that when memories get fuzzy later down the road, you remember exactly when you wrote these points. I always write the dates next to my journal entries and it always amazes me to look back and see what I wrote back then, how I felt, etc.

What I have now that makes me feel abundant:

Going Through Hard Times

It can be hard to stay positive and think abundance when you are going through hard times. Sometimes very hard. Here are some things that may help you feel better when you are going through hard times:

- Take a walk in nature
- Listen to music that makes you feel good
- Create something that is meaningful to you
- Read a wonderful book
- Buy yourself flowers or a treat that is meaningful to you
- Watch something on tv that is merry-making
- Engage in prayer and talking to God, unloading on Him

- Remember and write down your already-experienced blessings
- Get involved with a fun activity that makes you feel better
- Remember that you are more than a conqueror in Christ
- Go back to the breath and take a deep breath of fresh air
- Watch a comedy show or a comedy performance and get laughing

In fact, I would even dare to say that even in the hardest times, we can not only turn to God for help, support and advice but we can also discover the things that make us happiest in those difficulties. A lady I was once ministering to told me that in the midst of one of the hardest times in her life, she stayed positive by focusing on her dogs and on going for long walks with her dog. Ultimately, she realized how happy being with her dogs made her and so she decided to leave her work and get involved with a new career that allowed her to be around dogs all the time. It was a wonderful transition for her, one that allowed her a much greater career happiness and one that may not have come around had she not gone through that exceptionally difficult time.

Another thing that was positive about ministering to this lady was that she was genuinely doing everything she could to stay positive and to be happy in the midst of her troubles. She would speak positively about herself, she would think positive thoughts, write herself sweet notes on the bathroom mirror, she would cook special meals for herself and create homemade meals for her dogs, and she focused on the things that made her happy. To that, I say good for her!

Dire Straits

A man I knew and who taught me a great deal was one who had dealt with difficulties all his life. He had had a very difficult life and he was working to be positive and to help himself out of his troubles. He had never grown up with much money and so he also had a negative view of money but still knew he had to work in order to make sure he had enough to support himself. What impressed me was his outlook on life. Even though he had been through some difficulties, he still managed to be positive, to be good to others, to treat people with kindness, to put his best into his work and to work hard for everything that came his way. This is exemplary behavior. What I found so incredible about this particular man's experience is that he used difficulties and parlayed them into his benefits. What I mean by this is that he ended up using the difficulties that he saw in the world and he began to think of ways of making things better for people. He felt that he had skills in the financial sector and instead of focusing and dwelling on what was negative, he ended up becoming a financial advisor for friends and for family and began to parlay his acquired knowledge and understanding of financial systems into being a phenomenal financial advisor, using Christian principles to help people make more of a return than some of the larger investment firms. While he didn't have much growing up and he didn't have positive examples around him, he used the skills that he did have and his love for learning to dig himself out of the financial hole he found himself in and that allowed him to work well with other people, helping them secure their own financial future. I find this example to be amazing because he could have gotten stuck and dwelled on the negatives and on all the disadvantages and unfairness that life had thrown his way; instead he decided to be positive, to work hard, not to allow his future to be dictated by the limitation of his past and to make a life for himself with a wonderful skill that he now knew very well.

The Reality of Being Positive

Being positive does not mean not facing reality. It means that we are positive, stay positive, speak positively over our lives and do our best to think positively. It means to know that God has helped us through things before (even some things you didn't know He had a hand in) and since He has helped us before, He will help us again. Being positive does not mean not making your payments and saying "God, You do everything" but praying to see how God can help you in any situation you are facing.

A mom of three I knew was struggling to make ends meet. Her three children needed help focusing in school and she was feeling overwhelmed, being the only breadwinner in the home. She prayed for help and sure enough, her local church decided to help her with child care duties by opening up a free day care facility, and provided her with some food supplies to help her make her meals. Her kids were also offered free peer tutoring and mentorship by other students who were in older grades and excelling in their studies. All of this happened because she prayed and because she expected wonderful breaks and good things to happen.

Another woman I had heard speaking had been praying for her daughter to return home because she had become a victim of human trafficking. She had prayed long and hard for her daughter to be released from her traffickers and that she would be returned safely to her home and would come back to Church. I will never forget the day I was sitting in the pew at Church and the fulfillment of this mom's prayer had happened: her daughter had returned home and she was back in Church. It took much doing but the mom and her husband had never given up hope. This was an example of a miracle and definitely the fruit of parental prayers, thinking with hope and keeping positive.

9

Expecting God's Best

Focusing on God's best means that we are believing for great things to happen to us, for us, and through us. God wants to give you his best and so when we stay positive and we stay in faith, we are opening the door to receiving His very best. You may be saying to yourself *"This is never going to work, I don't have the right education, the right connections, I didn't come from the best family."* But none of that matters. When God decides to bless you, He isn't looking to what others say about you to make the final choice, the final decision. He is looking to your heart and to your faith. He knows you better than anyone and so when He counts you in, it doesn't matter what others say.

A friend was once telling me how they had applied to a job as an engineer but the job was out of town and he didn't have the money to travel there. He knew he was qualified for the job and he knew that he could do the job - he had the skills necessary. He just didn't have the money to get there but he decided to apply anyway, to try his luck. He prayed that if this was in fact God's will, that He would make a way for him to be the successful applicant. He prayed that God would inspire him to provide superior answers to the interview questions and that someway or other, that he would be the applicant with the best responses and ultimately, the candidate selected. Fast forward two months later, and the company decided to hire him for the job because they were so impressed with his online application and with all his responses. They paid for him to move to the location where the job was, with full salary and benefits and very generous stipend for all expenses. The man got down on his knees and thanked God sincerely for bringing him this career-changing opportunity and for making him the successful applicant. He found out later that the company had had a record number of applicants but that his genuine, kind, positive and caring attitude is what made the difference for them!

Getting Up Each Morning with Expectation

Many people get up each day and they either expect nothing to happen or they expect bad things to happen. Instead, try getting up in the morning and saying *"Lord, I know You are going to bring me something wonderful today!"* And be in expectancy about that.

God hears every prayer we make whether out loud or in our minds. We would be well to realize that He loves us very much and wants the best for us. But we must activate that goodness, those blessings, those good breaks. So when we say to ourselves *"God, I know that You are going to bring me Your best and You are going to help me be successful today. What do I have to do today?"* When we do that, we are not only showing our dependence on Him but we are also activating His goodness and His blessings in our lives.

Many people go through each day not activating God's wonderful goodness and not praying. God looks to do wonderful things in all our lives and waits for us to come and to pray to Him so that He can do fantastic things in their lives. The trick is to pray for it and to activate it. If we don't do that, God will not move on our behalf.

A friend of mine whom I will call Julia grew up an atheist and when she discovered that I was a praying Christian, she told me early on how surprised (actually she used the word shocked) she was that prayer is defined as a two-way conversation. Prayer is meant to be a conversation where God also explains, guides and helps us. She had said that she could feel and sense that God was trying to do wonderful things in her life but that she hadn't been praying for any of the good things she wanted to see. I gently suggested we try to pray together and for her to at least see if anything would happen. She was amenable and began to see things shifting and moving in the direction she had been praying for. She then came to a roadblock - something that was posing her a significant challenge. I advised her to pray through the problem and the roadblocks and to see herself being successful through them. She began to do so and began to see things, again, moving in the right direction.

Expecting God's Best

Expecting God's best means:
* waking up each day thanking God for His blessings and the things you already have
* knowing that if we stay positive and stay in faith, we will come to see His new blessings come to pass
* helping us see that we may have one idea for ourselves but that God may have better ideas for us
* having faith that God will do amazing things that surpass your expectations
* knowing that if we keep praying, we will come to see the realization of the best things
* knowing that He is bringing us His best, not just what we think is the best

Here is an image that I have come to see as being very meaningful:

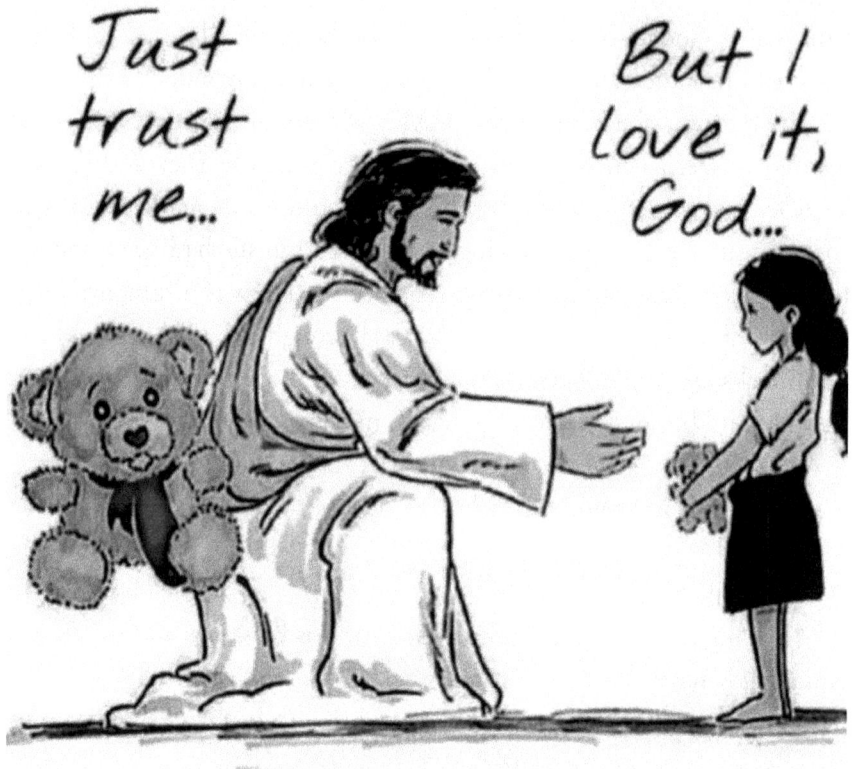

The little girl loves her teddy bear and it clearly means something to her - we all have things in our hands that mean something to us. Jesus has something better for her and given that He is Jesus (and He knows better than us), He is letting her know that He has better for her. The little girl (just like us) may be having a hard time letting go of her possession, but she is being encouraged to trust in God that He has better. We also see that Jesus is bending down, coming down to her level in order to talk to her, in order to let her know that He has better. That is very telling because God always comes to us right where we are - we don't need to be "perfect" or this way or that, we can come to Him as we are and we are encouraged to do so. He will meet us wherever we are and however we are.

Ask God About It....Don't Rely On Your Own Understanding

A woman I knew was about to get married to a man. She was nuts about him and she couldn't wait to marry him. She would walk around the office, excitedly talking about him, planning their wedding and had gotten pregnant from him. Her family and friends said that they were pleased with her choice to marry him and that she wanted to marry him. They said that he seemed great on all fronts and really seemed to care about her.

All the signs seemed to be pointing "green light", go ahead. The man seemed great. He certainly seemed to check off all the right boxes. One thing that this girl did not do is to ask God if this was the right man for her. A person can seem great but you have to take it to God before you take it to anyone else. Immediately after they got married, the man became very lazy, chose not to work despite having had a top-level degree and began verbally abusing their young daughter. From the time the baby arrived, the man refused to work to support his family, he berated his wife and when she was old enough, he began to verbally abuse the daughter. This was clearly not the man for her and he clearly needed help.

What am I saying? We need to ask God for His input, His best. We need to consult with the One who knows each person's heart and to find out what He is saying, not just what your family and friends are saying. In Scripture, there are many times when people were deceived into believing something that ended up not being true because they didn't ask God or because they didn't heed what He was saying. He is the only One who knows everything and sees everything so we would be wise to seek His counsel for anything we do.

Faith Is the Currency of Heaven

It is not need that gets God to move. It is faith. Faith is what pushes God to act on our behalf. In the Bible, we see time after time how people demonstrated faith and were healed, were saved, were helped and were blessed because they believed in God's promises and did as He led them to do.

Having faith is also a way of saying *"I trust You, God. I know You have my best interests at heart and while I may not initially or immediately understand what You're doing, I believe in Your goodness and I believe You will do Your best for me."* That is very powerful. That is surrender. It is what tells God that you are willing to trust in Him, lay your faith in Him, and let Him show you the best way.

Faith is also a synonym for hope and when we come to God, we can always have hope because nothing is impossible for Him. Literally, not one thing.

Answers to Frequently Asked Questions

Over the years, friends, family and people I have ministered to have asked me some of the following questions so I thought it would be very helpful to have them here, as a handy tool to help better understand God.

Q: Can we pray to have more faith?

A: Certainly. It would be wise to do so. We can pray for anything, so why not that? When we pray to have increased faith, we pray for a greater amount of trust in God and we receive it. He wants us to believe in Him so when we pray to Him for more faith, He will always answer that prayer.

Q: *Is it necessary to read Scripture and why?*

A: Reading Scripture is extremely important because it teaches you about the personality and ways of God, it explains human nature and wisdom, it shows us the miracles God has performed, it explains to us what God's will is and looks like, it shows us the power of prayer, and much more. Reading Scripture each day is intended to bring happiness, understanding, insight, wisdom and essentially, brings us into a closer relationship with God. The Bible contains all the promises of God so when we read it, we can see the good things He wants for us. Don't judge a book until you've read it.

Q: *How do we know when something is God's will?*

A: He will make it clear if you ask. If you ask if this is the right job for me and you don't get it, that's one way He will answer. If you ask for His will, He will always tell you, either directly, through another person, somehow or other, He will get the answer to you. He is waiting to be asked.

Q: *Can I pick and choose what I want to believe in Scripture?*

A: Scripture is all of the inerrant Word of God. It is all inspired by Him and there are no mistakes in it, nor has anything been left out. As such, we need to take it all as fact and I can tell you that God is perfect and does not make mistakes, so we need to take everything in the Word as factual, not choose what we want to take and leave what we don't want, like a salad bar. The Word is also a really effective way of getting to know the personality of God, including what He allows and doesn't allow.

Q: If I pray for something, will I for sure get it?

A: Not necessarily. You see, we may see something as great or ideal to have but we don't see the full picture. As such, we could be asking for something that may ultimately not be the best for us. God knows what's best all the time, and as such, He will bring us His best. Sometimes (as has been my experience) he will give us something that we asked for just to show us how it wasn't all we thought it was going to be. One thing to keep in mind, though, is that if He doesn't bring us exactly what we asked for, He will bring us better.

I am going to illustrate this last point a bit further: A girl I will name Tamar got married in hopes of having a happy life. She thought she was making the right decision and married a certain man. After the wedding, he started acting very roughly with her. She told me about how one night, he tried to choke her. Right away, she packed her bags and left. This young woman had gotten married in the hopes of having a happy life with this man but all she got was a horrible man who clearly didn't treat her correctly. She became a little bit depressed and struggled to get back out there to meet a new possible, suitable mate. One day, a family friend suggested a young man that he knew of that might be a suitable fit. He had everything going for him. After much hesitation, they decided to meet over coffee and talk. Today, they have been married for two years and are expecting their first together.

Trust in God, seek Him and His ways. Grow your relationship with Him. You are going to need Him every step of the way, and that's not a bad thing!

10

You Are A Magnet....What Are You Calling Forth?

We are all like magnets. We call forth what we think about, speak and put our focus on. And when we speak positive, faith-affirming words like "*I know I am coming together with the love of my life*" or "*I am excited because I am getting into the university of my dreams*", we are indicating to God that we have faith in Him and that we want to see come alive on earth that which we know is in our heart.

When we say negative words like "*It's hopeless, I am never going to get this done*" or "*What's the point, my child is too far gone*", those are excellent recipes for stopping and hindering your blessings. Speaking life and faith-affirming words increases your magnetism to the good things. Speaking death and doubt-affirming words decreases your magnetism to the bad things. Which one do you want to call forth today?

Practice

It can be difficult to focus on always saying positive things and to eliminate the negative things from our vocabulary. But this is an important practice to get into because our words are very important and our words are what attract and bring in good things into our lives. If we don't take the time to speak positively and to act positively, then we cannot expect for the positive to show up in our lives.

A woman that I know well always spoke negative words over her life and was always saying how old she was and how she was feeble, that she was in her last days. I told her exactly what I am telling you today: speak the things that you would like to appear in your life and leave out those things that you don't wish to appear in your life. Unfortunately in the case of this woman, she did not listen to my warnings and as time progressed, I saw the negative effects that her words were taking in her life and on her life and in the life of her husband. I began to see how she started to look old and started to feel like she was unable to do many things. She wasn't changing the channel and thinking and speaking positively over the things that she wanted to see and as such, she was seeing only negative things coming up and bringing negative things into her life.

We need to realize how powerful our words and our thoughts are and how they change the course of our lives. The words you speak and the thoughts you engage can also make you feel good or they can make you feel defeated. Again, **the negative thoughts and the negative words may come to your consciousness but it's important to choose carefully what you accept into your consciousness and into your vocabulary!**

> The negative thoughts and the negative words may come to your consciousness but it's important to choose carefully what you accept into your consciousness and into your vocabulary!

You Are a Child of God

Many people go through life feeling defeated, like they aren't going to get anywhere in life. Those people are actually attracting bad luck, and bad breaks. I know one man that I had previously ministered to who would speak just about no positive words over his life. Listening to him, you'd think that he was the most miserable man on earth. He had a lovely home, children who loved and respected him, a little bit of money in the bank, parents who loved him and one of the best senses of humor you could ever hope to find in a person, and some health. He was a regular riot but his words were self-defeating and self-deprecating. He kept insisting that everything was hard, that the cards were all stacked against him, that he didn't believe good breaks could happen to him and that life was just too hard. In his old age, those things one by one came true. All of those negative things he was speaking over himself had come to pass, one by one, and things were not getting better.

When I was ministering to him, I tried to remind him to be positive, to speak well over himself and to stop putting himself down. Unfortunately, he wasn't having any of it. He didn't change his attitude. That was about three years ago as of this writing and things have only deteriorated since.

You don't need to struggle so hard. You don't need to suck up so that people will throw you a crumb. What you do need to do is stay in faith, work hard at your job and at everything God tells you to do and you will see good favor and good things come to you. Like a magnet, you will attract good breaks, good fortune and all the best. Just stay in faith and it will come to you.

Speaking those positive words over yourself and thinking those positive thoughts over yourself will always help you attract good things and bring those good things into your life more quickly.

It's Not About Once or Twice

Speaking positive words and thinking positive thoughts both need to be daily habits. They are not things that you can only do once or twice if you want to see results. They need to be regular habits you do daily. If that means that you take a specific time each day to do so or you put reminders to do so in your phone or calendar or what have you, then do that. You need to get into the regular habit of speaking and thinking positively over yourself and your life.

"Why is this important, Christine?"

I liken this process to a rock that needs to move from here to there. Saying "move" once to the rock will not be enough. No. You need to speak to the rock each day and move it a little bit each day for it to have permanent effects.

Also, it takes some time for the positive thoughts and words to get into your subconscious. It takes time for the thoughts and words to be ingrained into you and so in order to see regular results, you will need to engage in this process again and again. Some people get into the practice of doing this 5-6 times a day and that's great.

What I have found works really well for me is to have a daily, morning reminder to do my prayers, meditation, visualization and speaking my positive words which I enjoy doing over my morning latte. That way, I know that I am setting up my day correctly.

The Role of Prayer

The role of prayer can also not be underestimated. When we pray to Jesus, we are praying to the most powerful Entity in the world. When we pray, we are stating our reliance on Him and on His power and we are saying "This is what I would like and what I feel God is guiding me to. Is this the right thing to want and if so, would You bring it to me? If it isn't the right thing to want, please speak to my heart and tell me."

Jesus always answers in one of three ways:

1. Yes and here you go.
2. Not yet but if you wait patiently and in thanksgiving, you will come to see it happen.
3. No, but I have better for you.

Prayer was always intended (and was created to be) a two-way conversation with God. One way would be that you are the only one speaking and God is listening. Two-way means that He listens and He responds to you. He may respond in one or more of several possible ways: you may get an idea or an impression, you may have an opportunity knocking on your door, a door may close to indicate to you that you will be receiving better or you may have a person come into your life to guide you further because there is more you need to know.

We are privileged to be able to pray. Yes, I said privileged. Why do I say that? Because when we pray, we are engaging the most powerful God (God Almighty) and we are stating our dependence on Him. According to my experiences, God does not disappoint and God does answer. So be on the lookout.

11

Strategy

One of the most important points I can make in this book is to talk to you about strategy. Strategy in life, love, and every area in-between. It is one of the most important things God has ever taught me: that there is a way and a strategy behind everything! The best part is: you don't have to figure out what the strategy is, He will tell you and He will guide you to it.

For example (I'll start with something small-ish), at the beginning of the covid pandemic, my cat was not dealing well. I also read that many animals were not dealing with their owner's lifestyle changes very well. He was having a very hard time adjusting to me being home and then me working from home, etc. He started attacking me and my family members. It was scary. Then the Lord helped me understand that the way I was relating to him had to change because the environment and circumstances had changed. I had to put up certain rules and boundaries and that even when I was home, I needed to instill space because he was seeing me too much.

The same is true for how I was to deal with the man of my life. I had to talk to him and deal with him in a certain way that made sense for him and for his love language. The Lord began to explain to me how this man (not all men) but this man needed to be talked to, what he valued most, what he didn't like and when he needed space or needed me to be around. I found our rapport changed completely for the better once I consistently instilled these changes and it was one of the most helpful realizations that I still use to this day.

Another example is how I was praying about my finances and realized that I was not being a good steward with some of my money. I was not investing it properly and it was just sitting there, not doing anything for me. I knew this needed to change, of course, and I was determined to do a better job stewarding my money because the Lord first trusts you with a little and then when He sees you being a good steward with a little, He trusts you with more. I don't know about you but I am hoping that He trusts me with more!

Here is that Scripture: (Luke 16:10-14)

"Whoever can be trusted with small things can also be trusted with big things. Whoever is dishonest in little things will be dishonest in big things too. If you cannot be trusted with worldly riches, you will not be trusted with the true riches. And if you cannot be trusted with the things that belong to someone else, you will not be given anything of your own. "You cannot serve two masters at the same time. You will hate one master and love the other. Or you will be loyal to one and not care about the other. You cannot serve God and Money at the same time."

Prayer, and meditation are both also part of the strategic process and are part of living a positive life that leads to abundance and to God's best. I know I have mentioned it earlier in the book but it's very important to take the time to pray and to meditate on what He is guiding us to do and how.

One of my Doctorate professors pointed this out to me very succinctly and she was right: every day you need to check-in with God to see what He wants you to do that day. It's the first conversation you need to have in your day because nobody knows better than Him and each day, He has specific things He wants you to do. He won't tell you on Tuesday what He wants you to do on Thursday, because His advice and counsel are time-released. He has a reason for not having told you yesterday and for waiting until today. It's also super important (remember this point from earlier) to ask clarification and probing questions to understand more and to get more details about what He wants us to do.

I realized fairly quickly that long ago, I knew that God had put the dream on my heart to be a published author of many, many books. During a bit of time I had off of work during summer and Christmas breaks, He reminded me of this promise and put some of Joel Osteen's books in my hands. He reminded me that I needed to get moving on writing those books and putting my best effort into the content of each book. Why? Because those books, sermons and audio programs helped and still do help me tremendously every time I am going through something. I would love to pay that forward and help someone else who could benefit from them!

I'd like to give you an opportunity now to think about certain strategies that have helped you in the past. Maybe they are strategies God has already given you and you implemented them and maybe you haven't yet implemented them. If you haven't asked or implemented yet, do so and jot down the results. This does not need to be done in 1 day or 1 week...results sometimes take a while to be realized but this is your starting point. If there isn't enough room on this page, please feel free to jot down this chart on your device, paper or journal and to configure the chart as you would like, so you have enough room to put in all the details.

Problem	Strategy	Result
-------	--------	------
-------	--------	------

Specific Ways = Specific Results

I did come to realize several years ago that there is a specific way of doing something that will lead to specific results and there is a definite way of doing things that will lead to negative results. We need to be incredibly mindful of the strategies that we use that will lead us to certain results because when we undertake the right strategies, we are setting ourselves up for total success! I realized that success may take a little bit of time but that every day and in every way that we take the right actions, we should see ourselves getting closer and closer to our final positive result that we were looking to achieve.

This is not just a concept for adults but also one for children, tweens, teens, young adults, etc. When your child is looking for help and for advice on how to handle something, you would be well to instruct them that there is a certain strategy that they will need to use to reach their goal and that they need to be consistent in taking the right actions that will lead them to the final results. Taking action for one or two or ten days is not enough. We all need to dedicate ourselves to undertaking those actions on a daily basis -- this will likely mean using our planners and agendas and calendars to help us keep track of our progress and to help us realize that we are taking steps, solid ones, toward the fulfillment of our goals and dreams! Using visual motivators is also a really good idea because those help us keep our eyes on the prize. For instance, many people use images of fit people when they are on the treadmill and doing workouts - it helps keep them going and remembering that they can do this and that even though it is hard, this is the body they are working towards.

Some people are naturally good at this (and that's great). And some people need a little more help in keeping this a consistent part of their lifestyle. I remember when I challenged myself to do some working out every day for 30 days and used a calendar to help me keep track. I did it consistently for about 10-15 days and then got lazy and started forgetting. I look back on the calendar now and see the gaps (the days where I did nothing...not even some yoga, for instance) and I use it as a reminder that I need to keep myself more accountable to my goals. That means that I will use a hard copy calendar, one on my phone, reminders and encouragement posted in my room and people to keep me on-task and motivated. It is not totally easy to get into the groove of sticking to something so new and so it makes sense that one would need aids like this.

Making Excuses

I say this with all the respect in the world: some people are great at making excuses and not following through. For example, I was having a conversation with someone and I mentioned how great it would be to have such-and-such (a very fit and sensational body) and that I had an example or two that I admired to emulate. Their response was along the lines of "Yes, but that person has private chefs, personal trainers, etc., etc." I don't actually subscribe to that line of thinking. We often think that celebrities have it so much easier than we do and that it's for reasons like they have more money, more this and more that, and so that's why they have better everything. Fact is, celebrities are people too and they can have just as many demands on their time as anyone else, not to mention that they often have 12-14 hour work days on production sets.

The fact is, you can make time and energy for something if it is important enough to you. There is always a way of getting something done and accomplishing our purpose. Of course, also having cheerleaders in your corner and people who are in the loop about what you're working hard to do and can keep you accountable is also great to have. When we really want something, we can and will find a way to accomplish it.

All Areas

At the beginning of this book, I mentioned that abundance relates to all areas of life, and it does. After all, we cannot be abundant if we just have money but we don't have our health, or we cannot be abundant if we just have wealth but our personal lives are in shambles. It is for this reason that this book focuses on all areas of life and all areas of abundance. In Scripture (Jeremiah 29:11), when God spoke about having plans for us "For I know the plans I have for you," declares the Lord, "plans to prosper you and not to harm you, plans to give you hope and a future," He was not only talking about wealth and money but wealth in all areas. So, let's pause for a moment and I'd like to invite you to think about how you're doing in all areas of your life.

Let's break it down by area and for each, write out how you feel you are doing. If necessary (and nothing wrong with it) write it out and then set it aside for a little while, coming back to it later and seeing and reviewing it with fresh eyes. If the categories mentioned here blend in together for your specific scenario, I invite you to take a journal or sheet of paper and write out all that you would like.

Areas (these are not written in any particular order):

Personal:

Professional:

Money:

Career:

Health:

Please feel free to add more categories as you see fit or feel inspired.

Now think about where you feel God is guiding you in those areas.

Said differently, take a moment to pray and meditate about each area and think about where God is guiding you to go for each area of your life. Here is a simple prayer you can use to help get you started with this:

"Lord, I would like to ask You how I am doing in each of these areas, for the purposes of improvement. You know me better than I know myself and so I ask You for Your input and wisdom on how I am doing in each area and how I can improve in each area. I thank You in advance for Your answers and Your wisdom. In Jesus' name. Amen."

I caution you not to think about things only in terms of status quo. Not at all. Where God leads He provides, so He is not looking at your current bank account and your current status. He is looking at things you may not yet see and setting you up for successes in life that you may not yet see a way to achieving.

Meditation & Relaxation How-To

Meditation is a wonderful way of calming your mind, and letting yourself be still for a few moments. It is a tremendously effective practice and one that you can do as many times as you would like in a day. It helps to calm the mind, to think more clearly, to be inspired, and to gain perspective on anything.

As some people may be new and, or inexperienced at meditation, here are some steps you could take in beginning or improving your meditation practice:

1. Find yourself a quiet place to meditate where you will not be interrupted
2. You can turn the lights off if you would like
3. Close your eyes as this will help you focus
4. You can use soft music in the background if that helps you
5. Clear your mind from any and all worries

6. Invite Jesus and the Holy Spirit to help you stay focused and to guide your meditation, to help you relax
7. Ask Jesus and the Holy Spirit to help guide your mind, thoughts and sensations to specific areas and things that you need to pay attention to
8. Keep your eyes focused on Jesus the entire time you are doing this. You can do this by imagining His name written in the sky or by imagining His heart loving you
9. When the Lord is showing you something, there is nothing wrong with asking for more information and for more details. Meditation, like prayer, is meant to be a two-way conversation
10. Breathe in deeply and enjoy the relaxation

If you feel you are getting answers or guidance during a meditation, that is wonderful. Feel free to jot it down after the meditation so you don't lose the thought. The release of perspective, calmness and much more are some of the many benefits to meditation.

Take my friend Janine, for example. She felt strongly that she was being guided to start a teaching ministry but the job and the resources she had at the time were not sufficient to get her there. Her work did not give her the time to dedicate to this the way it needed and she had extraordinary payments to make given some personal problems she had encountered a few years ago. Well, the Lord knew all of this and lo-and-behold, He changed her life. Circumstances and challenges that were in her life started moving out of her way quickly, as she began to take the first and then second, and then third and so on and so forth to accomplish what God had put on her heart. Janine got to see God's great work in her life and she saw her life completely changed once she started taking the first steps and having faith in what God was guiding her to do.

Making Mistakes

One of the questions I am asked most often when I am ministering to people is: *"What if I make a mistake? What if I mess up? What if I don't do this step or that one correctly? Will I miss my whole destiny? Will God stop loving me? Will I be forever condemned for one wrong move?"*

The short answer is: no, God will not condemn you, will certainly not stop loving you, you will not miss your whole destiny and you will have opportunities to fix and to correct where you went wrong.

Not to worry.

God has already factored in that we are all human: creatures that make mistakes and do things incorrectly. As such, He makes provisions for us and helps us get back on track even when we do make those mistakes. He is fantastic at forgiving us for wrong steps and wrong moves because what He looks at is our heart. What does that mean? He looks at our heart and He looks at the fact that we are trying, and He provides opportunities to fix things and just like a GPS, to recalculate and have another chance to get it right.

God is a God of second and third and fourth chances. I don't know anyone (myself included) who hasn't made lots of errors and has needed helpful supplies of God's good grace, love and patience to help us all through. Also, a special note to anyone who might feel like "less than" for messing up and needing His good grace: you are NOT less than, God loves you just as much today as He did any other day and He does not keep score of your mess-ups. If you mess up or messed up, you just repent for it and you move forward in the way He tells you to. It may take some extra time to get back on track and to fix things so that you can get back on track, but there is always a way (with God) to get back on-track and to fix things.

Going back to a friend of mine, who did mess up on part of what she was supposed to do. She went left instead of right and as a result, she found herself in a space where she wasn't supposed to be. I told her the same thing that I am telling you: acknowledge it and move forward. The trick is not to get stuck in self-loathing, self-deprecation and seeing only the negative. That is not what is going to get you further along and it is not what God wants for you. Move forward toward the fruitful outcome you know you are supposed to be working toward.

> **The trick is not to get stuck in self-loathing, self-deprecation and seeing only the negative. That is not what is going to get you farther along and it is not what God wants for you.**

When I did make those mistakes, one thing in particular that I found helpful is asking God for patience. I knew that my mistake had set me back and it was getting me really frustrated. So, I decided that I would pray for more patience and for the presence of mind to go back, and this time, to do things the way that He says to do them. I have been a happier camper because of it and have seen things move forward far more quickly than I could have anticipated.

It is a great idea for you to also ask for this grace, peace, extra patience and more too. I once heard someone say that because that person is a man or woman of God, that God will help them more and love them more. Not true at all. God loves us all the same and He longs for you to turn to Him, no matter how badly you have messed up in the past, no matter how far down the proverbial rabbit hole you have gone, no matter any and all of it. God still loves you and He remains at the ready to help you and to move you forward to all that He has called you to be.

Showing Grace, Love and Understanding To One Another

People need people to show them grace, love and understanding. We are all trying, we will all, at some point, mess up and we need and require others to be kind, caring and wonderful about our mess-ups. This means that we don't talk negatively behind each others' backs, we are and remain supportive and when we can, we help. I am a firm believer that if we did these things, we would all be much better off as a society and as a result. This means that instead of kicking someone when they are down (knocking them further down), we can, instead, lend a helping hand. We can provide helpful encouragement. We can provide stories of how we were once down and we got better. We would tell them these things for the purposes of helping them feel loved and supported.

Taking this a step further, when children, tweens and teens see adults (anywhere and everywhere) demonstrate this kindness and caring to one another, they take example and for many, it prompts and propels them to do a good deed to someone else. The younger generation takes note of what we are doing and when they see good examples, they begin to emulate them.

I remember seeing an elderly lady with grocery bags who was having trouble getting the bags into her home. A young boy who was nearby in the neighborhood saw that she was struggling and asked his teacher if he could be excused for a minute to go help her. The teacher noted his kind thoughts and intentions and kept an eye on him while he went to go help the elderly lady. **Such small acts of kindness on behalf of anyone and everyone can go such a long way in helping us all be happier and healthier.** I would imagine the good feelings of joy that young man had when he helped the elderly lady with her groceries. There may have been many other people in the area (including his classmates) who may have seen this young man's act of kindness and may have been enticed to do a kind act for someone else in another time and another place.

It's no different when we are adults. We need to be kind, loving, warm and supportive to one another. Even if it is a person you may feel you dislike and who has not been kind to you in the past. You never know how your act of kindness may change them. This will certainly go a long way in making sure you are demonstrating God's best and that you are being good to His children, something God always loves.

How can we show grace, love and understanding to one another? Here are some suggested ways:

- Compliment someone in their efforts for self improvement
- Remind someone that they are on their way and to commend them for taking the first steps to betterment
- Talk to someone about the power of prayer and how we can always turn to God for extra helpings of love, grace and patience
- When someone is going through a hard time, bring them something wonderfully comforting and let them know that you are there for them to talk
- Be that shoulder to cry on
- Remind them and commend them on the fact that they are improving a little every day
- When someone messes up, share a comforting story about how you once messed up too, for the purpose of letting them know they are not alone in their mess-up
- When someone is down, remind them that Jesus is always there to pick them up and help them back up. God's love, grace and mercy are endless.
- Make provisions for someone's mess up and tell them it's ok

I won't forget when one day, I was quite late for work and I was on the highway in stalled traffic. I came to the inevitable realization that I was never going to make it on time and that I clearly hadn't left myself enough time to get to the location, given the two car accidents that were on route. I was sitting in my car on the driveway (not even inching along) and squirming, decided to text the person and let them know I was running late. I was frankly afraid at how they were going to react and respond . To my astonishment and pleasant surprise, the text came back immediately, and the person said "Not to worry. Just be safe." My heart actually melted a little. I was very touched by the response because I was worried about how they were going to respond. This is an excellent example of how this (relative) stranger extended grace, kindness and courtesy to me and how it literally warmed my heart when they did!

When we extend such kindness, grace and courtesy to others, we definitely feel good. We may not always get the feedback from the person to know how the grace we extended made them feel at that moment, but we can definitely surmise that we have extended this kindness to people in the past and that in itself should make us feel good.

Constructive Criticism

Now, when I say to show kindness and caring to others, it does not mean that we cannot provide them with helpful constructive criticism. We certainly can, when the person is ready and open for it. What do I mean by that? If the person is asking for feedback, then they have to be open to some constructive criticism, and you can kindly and gently tell them where they need to improve. This benefits the person tremendously because they will get to hear another person's take on things, and how they can improve their work and their output.

I always find it helpful to remind people that when you go to someone for constructive criticism, they are going to tell you about things that need to be improved and that need to be tweaked. There is nothing wrong with that and if you need some time to let it sit while you process the information, you can tell them that. The reason I make this point is that many people out there get angry (sometimes even enraged) when other people mention areas of improvement that they asked for, but they don't take the feedback well. (Of course, I've been there too). The best thing you can do in that case is to sit with the information a little and think it over, asking yourself the following questions:

1. Did this person give me constructive criticism with the best of intentions?
2. Did this person approach me thoughtfully and kindly?
3. Did this person have a point in what they were saying?
4. Will implementing this constructive criticism make my work better and therefore, should their input be implemented?

You may come to see after a little time that the person really did have your best intentions at heart and they were coming from a great place - a place where they are helping you to improve. If you feel it was not, then (as we all have free will) you can exercise your option to dismiss that piece of criticism and choose to move on from it without implementing it.

> **When we are working on self-improvement, we have to keep in mind that this will require work, this will require time and it will require patience. As such, we have to make sure that we are taking this in stride.**

Don't Just Jump In....Ask!

Not everyone is looking for constructive feedback all the time, so before we attempt to provide it, let's ask them if it's the right time or the right context for it. You could have the best of intentions, but if the person isn't ready to hear it, then it will fall on deaf ears or even worse, you may receive backlash. So don't just jump in, ask them if it's appropriate, and if it's a good time.

Most of the time (I have found), people need to mentally prepare for what they refer to as "negative feedback". They brace themselves for it in a way that indicates that they are about to receive the worst information in the world. That isn't necessary. Constructive feedback is your opportunity to grow and to get better, and while that does sometimes sting a bit, we need to keep in mind the overall good intent: that the person is gently, kindly and in a supportive way trying to help us improve.

So go ahead and ask and wait patiently for that answer. It may not be the best time but if the person can see you have good intentions, they will set time aside to hear you and your ideas out.

12

Getting God's Help....Do We Need It?

We definitely need God's help to accept, and to internalize feedback, not to mention to accept and to internalize His guidance. He always guides with the best of intentions, getting us to exactly where we need to be, and in the time frame that we need. There are set times for this and we don't always know when those times will be. God does and again, He knows the best times to get us all to where we need to be in the right time frame (not necessarily our time frame).

I will never forget when I got negative feedback at work about something I had done. I didn't realize that I had done something incorrectly, and when I got the negative feedback, I was not happy. I took it pretty hard and had to spend time with God in order to seriously think and reflect on the feedback. Once I realized that God was lovingly convicting me, I realized that there was also a realization of space to get better and to improve in the very area I had fallen short. When we pray and ask for His guidance and to reveal shortcomings, mess-ups, etc., we need to be thankful and then we need to take steps to make things right.

Making things right may be as simple as one apology, but it may not. The offense may be something that might take days, weeks, or even months or years to fix, but if we are serious about making things right, then we will pray for patience and for clarity of insight, and we will go ahead and do whatever is needed to make the situation right. Making things right is a process and while we may want the instant "happy" result, that may not be the reality we come to experience.

I was speaking to my friend about an area where she had made a mistake and gently, when the time was right, mentioned the error to her. I tried to include evidence of why that choice was a mistake and how she can fix it. She did see that there was a bit of an error on her part, but she had made the decision that she would not take the time to fix it. She stated that it would take too long and that she wasn't sure she wanted to put that much time, energy and effort into that endeavor. I tried to get her to understand that, in this case, the mistake was one that was made over many years and that it wouldn't take ten minutes to fix it but that with mindful and consistent actions, she could begin making reparations and fixing it a little each day.

Readers, I tell you this to impress upon you that while things may take time (certainly getting good at our walk with and relationship with Jesus is going to take lots of time) that it is time well worth spending. Why? Because in order to access His best for us, we need to have a solid relationship with Him because that is how He will guide us to His very best for us, better than we can see for ourselves. But you have to take the first steps, if you have not already done so.

Before I became a committed Christian, a friend told me that exact lesson and I didn't understand it. I couldn't fathom that and I was prepared to ask why this was important and how this was beneficial to me, to all of us.

Until I saw and experienced it myself.

I started praying for God to open my eyes and to show me how His will was wiser, smarter, better than mine. He started showing me that in personal matters, career, finances, business, essentially every area, how He guides to better. I was starting to see and experience how my own viewpoint was so darn limited and limiting and how His ways were better. Yes, I was at the time actually arrogant enough to think (initially) that my way and ways were better than His.

I won't forget how I prayed for a certain thing....here is that recount: I was serving on the board of Directors of a condo corporation and there was another board member who was also serving and with whom I was clashing. He and I were not seeing eye-to-eye, in fact our individual ways were diametrically opposite. Meeting after meeting I sat there, clashing with this man and obviously not enjoying it. He didn't seem to be enjoying it either. Instead of asking God what I should be doing, I went ahead and started praying on my own for him to step down from the board position. This was unwise because even when your prayer is answered, you don't know what else is lurking around the corner, so you really should ask for His take and His insight on the matter. Well, I didn't do that in this case and sure enough, one day very unexpectedly, this board member quit and stepped down. His decision was effective immediately. At the time, I was a bit happy about it, thinking that now I had a better opportunity to have things done for the betterment of the condo corp owners and in a different way than was being done in the past.

Well that's not what happened.

As that board member stepped down, another one came to the mic (figuratively speaking). He was even more forcefully making decisions and having his own ways met and basically began ruling with a proverbial iron fist. On top of it, he began berating me and putting me and my input down every chance he got. That's just not appropriate or business-like. It was a bad clash and was resulting in things becoming even worse than before. Had I asked, God would have told me a better way to handle things and a better, more strategic thing to pray for.

We definitely need God's help because we may not only not realize the full picture of things but we also need to ask for wisdom on how to deal with things in the right ways. He sees all of that and He knows how to help us navigate things but we need to ask him and then obey what He says, even if it doesn't make sense to us right away.

13

"But God Isn't Around & Doesn't Know Me"

Many people I talk to (of all different religions and different walks of life) regularly say to me that they don't know or want to believe in God because they don't know Him, He isn't "around" and they have no idea about the personality of God.

I understand where they are coming from because I, too, was like that. I didn't know God either until I spent about a concentrated year spending time alone with Him, reading Scripture, reading testimonials from people, and listening regularly to different sermons. Just as it takes time to get to know a new person who may become a good friend or a best friend, God is no different. He has a certain, set personality and He wants you to have a relationship with Him. I'll say that again because this is a really important point: **He wants you to have an active, living, breathing, vibrant relationship with Him.**

One of the most lovely things I learned in my closeness with God since I began many years ago is that it is a living, active, vibrant relationship and in the same breath, yes, God does know who you are, loves you infinitely more than you can ask or imagine and frankly, knows every hair on your head (Luke 12:7). You, like me, may not have been conscious of having an active relationship with Him but He has been conscious of you and knows you very well. Scripture says that He knew you in your mother's womb and if you read my first book, Jesus Loves You, you will see that He knew you before you were created and loved you deeply from then.

So, what does a living, active and vibrant relationship mean? It means that like your best friend, you can and should literally talk to Him every day, share your thoughts and ideas, feelings, etc., including asking questions, asking for explanations, insight and more. He is there and whether you need to unload or show your happiness or any range of emotion, He is there to talk to you at 2 in the afternoon and at 2 in the morning. He is always there and ready and available and it's great because once you begin to understand the wisdom that exists and can permeate into every decision you make (if you allow it) you will see how your life can improve.

Too often in society, we don't teach and we don't talk about how people need to be close to God. We don't talk about it in schools, and we don't really actively talk about it in various social circles. When I was young, I had never been to a Church that talked about the active and vibrant relationship available with Christ. I learned about it in later years through a friend who had a very active relationship with Him. I truly feel that this lack of going to God is one of the biggest (if not the biggest) reasons that peoples' mental health is deteriorating and that people are not taught to fight using Scripture and with the authority we have in Christ.

Some friends and family members asked me to outline the benefits that are available through a relationship with Christ and so I thought I would share them here, for the benefit of all you lovely readers:

* being able to talk and to converse with God at any time of the day, whether through your own mind or out loud via spoken word

* access to the greatest Mind in the world
* access to the greatest Wisdom in the world
* peace and unsurpassed happiness because you got things off your chest that were bothering you
* a plethora and abundance of resources to help you with every step of your own walk with Him
* the ability to show Him just how in-need of Him you are and just how vulnerable you are
* peace and unsurpassed happiness because you know that according to Scripture, you do whatever you can and then you leave it up to Him to help you through it
* knowing your Best Friend is there for you at any time
* knowing that your Best Friend can make anything happen at any time (and is not limited to the laws of the natural world)
* having His supernatural guidance through all of life's choices and decisions
* knowing that, no matter what kind of life you had or have, He loves you more than any human and He is always there, even if maybe your own parents or whomever weren't there for you
* access to the wisest of all books, the Bible, and being able to pray to the Holy Spirit (who lives right inside of you) for greater insight to better understand the Bible
* the knowledge that the disciples were ordinary men and yet, God did great things through them (I don't know about you, but I'm as ordinary as they get)

These are just some of the benefits to a life in an active relationship with Christ but the most important thing of all is to actually experience it. You have to actually start with step 1 and experience what that relationship is truly like.

Journal Keeping

Another recommendation I have is to keep a journal. Keeping a journal where you can write all your thoughts, feelings, prayers and more is a great way to keep track of things and to look back one day and see your progress. You will look back on your journals and you will feel better seeing the progress you have made to get to where you currently are in life and you will enjoy and appreciate the feelings of knowing that you have done such and such to improve your life.

Any kind of journal will do. I tend to prefer ones where there is Scripture or a daily devotional included on each page, helping to spur me and encourage me to read and remember Scripture as I go.

Journal Keeping with Your Spouse or Significant Other

A really nice idea is to have one journal for you and maybe one with your spouse or significant other. Why do I say this? Because it's a really nice thing to share your innermost thoughts and feelings with your partner and to come back to them later on and to see how you have both learned, experienced and grown over the years. Sharing that with your spouse or significant other will allow you both to feel much closer to each other and will allow you to share something really meaningful, not to mention be a party to each other's lives and growth as individuals and as a team.

Being a partner (whether spouses, boyfriend and girlfriend, fiances, whatever) means that that person gets to see and experience your innermost being, your soul. I always find it amazing when people say that they don't feel that they know their spouse that well because they haven't shared, whether that means sharing their thoughts, feelings, desires, whatever. Your spouse and, or your significant other is supposed to be that person with whom you can share your innermost thoughts and desires, feelings and secrets and have them be loving, kind and accepting of all you have shared. Having that shared journal is a great idea for having that relationship develop and become much deeper and more meaningful.

If you are one of those people that is feeling shy or nervous to begin that journey, know that you are not alone. So many people would feel that way and it takes a certain leap of faith to let the other person in, especially if it's not something you have ever done before or not something you have done for some time. Give yourself permission to take it one step at a time, one shared page (if you will) at a time and learn to let that person in, if God says it's the right person and the right time.

You will notice in this book that I always go back to that : ask God. Ask Him everything, share everything. He already knows you better than you know yourself and loves you with all your faults, flaws, insecurities and more.

It does also have to be said here and I would be remiss if I didn't point out the fact that if your spouse or significant other is not loving and kind and supportive of what you are going through, then that could be a problem. If your sharing is met with anything less than appreciation, kindness and support, then friend, I'm not sure that's the right relationship for you. Even if our partner is a wisecracking, joking, and generally a bit of a tougher person (which is fine), they still need to be loving and supportive of your feelings and ideas because that's what a healthy relationship requires. If yours is not, please pray to see what God would have you do in that situation.

14

Feeling Great & Taking Care...Mentally

Abundance definitely includes health, wellness and feeling great and that's why I want to dedicate this chapter and the next to feeling great and taking care. Chapter 14 will deal with feeling mentally great and taking care, while the following will deal with feeling physically great and taking care.

Taking care mentally means being really good to ourselves and giving ourselves the space to talk things out, to feel happy, to take breaks from work in order to rejuvenate and to do things that help us feel mentally at our best. It takes a lot of mental stamina to work at our best each day and so we need to be sure that we take time to unplug, to work out, to talk to our loved ones, to write (if you are so inclined) and to do activities that help our mental wellness and help us unburden. When we feel tired and overwhelmed, we are no longer working at our best or being our best for our family and friends and it doesn't matter who you are, taking breaks for your mental wellness is supremely important.

Here are some things that are known to help people feel mentally better. Try one or many. The point is that the goal is to feel better and more mentally fit and ready to take on life:

* work out
* meditation and yoga
* physical intimate activities
* talk things out or write things out
* watch something funny or relaxing
* read something funny or relaxing
* buy yourself flowers or something that makes you happy
* go for a walk in nature
* listen to classical music or music you find uplifting
* call a friend
* read a happy book
* do something nice for someone
* build something
* play an instrument
* attend a class or a reading
* pray
* drink water or tea or a cup of hot cocoa
* enjoy a coffee with a pal
* watch a movie
* take a nap
* take a nice, long shower or bubble bath
* watch a stand-up comedy show

Our mental health is so important and frankly, fragile. Something that happens in our day can set us off or can put us in a bad mood and it can take hours or days or more to make us feel better. This is why we need to find little ways of making ourselves happy, a little each day. When you take time to invest in your own mental health, everyone around you (not just family and friends but everyone) will find themselves enjoying your company more. Happiness is infectious because people love being around other people who make them happy and therefore, make their mental health a priority.

I once read that meditating for 15 minutes in your day is sufficient.

I don't know about you but I find the need to meditate a few times per day for those few minutes or for longer. It makes me calm my mind and my body so I can think more clearly and I can make the best decisions and be the best version of me. If I don't take that time (as many others can also attest to), we can find ourselves being cranky, short-tempered, irritable, annoyed and annoying and sometimes in the extreme, we can lash out at others. It takes honest self-reflection to come to the realization that you may need some help or you may need to slow things down a bit if you sense that you're getting to a point that isn't great.

Take a moment right now and do some guided meditation and relaxation, where you allow your mind to get calm, and at the end, why not jot down some ideas on how taking that time allowed you to feel, what you experienced, how it helped you and if something else or a modification next time can help you feel even better next time. I will provide a suggested guided meditation scenario and you are of course free to use it if you find it helpful. It may be a good idea to get to a quiet space where there are no interruptions while doing this exercise, to get the most out of the experience.

Suggested Guided Meditation: Imagine that you are alone, dressed in your most comfortable clothes, walking slowly and gingerly through a beautiful, tree-lined private, grassy area and it is just you and your thoughts. Everything here is happy and beautiful and exactly as you would like it to be. Ask the Holy Spirit to include anything else in the scenario that He will know you will need. Everything here is peaceful and happy and effortless and you enjoy the peaceful, gentle music or the total quiet that exists here. Time stands still here...there are no deadlines, no appointments....it is just you and relaxation. It is a beautiful, happy space and a place for you to go to explore your innermost happiness and comforting thoughts. Remember that in this space, there are no faults, no problems, everything is just happy all the time. The weather is perfect and exactly as you like it and you can sit, stand, wander around....the space is yours to feel happy and calm within and to move around as you like. Enjoy your time in this space and capture your happiness in this space.

When you have opened your eyes, write down (jot notes, whatever you want) a bit about how it helped, how you feel, etc.:

_____

We need to invest in our mental health each and every single day. I say this knowing, understanding and respecting how busy and full people's lives often are. We have demands coming at us, requests, people needing things, etc. I get it. But if we don't take time for our own mental wellness and well-being, we are not being the best version of ourselves for anyone.

Make a plan today to invest a bit of time each and every day into your own personal mental health practices and grab your journal, phone, calendar, whatever to make sure you make this a part of your daily practices and routines. If you start to get people around you who are noticing that positive changes are coming from these practices, that's wonderful. Write about it in your journal....it will make for a nice memory and possibly a benchmark for future mental health time. Said differently, peoples comments can help you see what is clearly working for you and can help you make it a regular, daily part of your life.

> **Investing in you and in your relationship with Christ is the best investment you can make.**

Investing in you and in your relationship with Christ is the best investment you can make. The returns will always be great and meaningful and who knows where your "you time" can ultimately lead.

In closing this chapter, I will give you a bit on how Adelaide, a lovely lady I know, took time to get into these practices for herself. She started off with just 10 minutes in the morning before she went off to work. She used some online classical music to calm her mind, connect to Jesus and overall, feel better. Through this meditation time, she also realized that her body was not feeling as strong as it needed to, so she decided to do good for herself and make it more of a priority to eat more healthy foods and to give herself the mental break after work that she knew she needed. She began giving herself more time to meditate because she saw how good it was feeling for her and she began to see how her mind and mental health were improving daily as a result. She wisely took the time to make it a part of her daily practice and slowly, began making more and more time for it in her day. She ended up deciding that this was causing her to be the best version of herself and chose to open up a meditation clinic that she could work on part time while also writing about the benefits of meditation and turning to Jesus through the Holy Spirit. You see, Adelaide also began experiencing a major reduction in the chronic headaches she had been experiencing previously and she was really enjoying playing classical music in the background so she decided to take up piano as well.

Now, I'm not saying you too will do these exact things, but what I am saying is that by taking the time to pray, meditate and visualize, we are tapping into the goodness of God and we are allowing ourselves to be taken on a wonderful journey of seeing what else He has in store for us. Won't you begin that journey today?

On to the physical health side of things....

15

Feeling Great & Taking Care...Physically

Our physical health is tremendously important and needs to be worked on a little each day. There are a myriad of things you can do each day to help you feel great and energized each day, being and feeling ready to take on the day. It's very simple...when you combine a healthy mind and you do all you have to do to ensure a healthy body, the results are an unstoppable you!

We all have so many things to do in our day and all of it is meaningful to us (otherwise I assume you wouldn't be doing it). But we also need to properly fuel our bodies to ensure that we are in the best position possible to do all we can do for our physical health.

> **God has created us to be whole and healthy but sometimes, we start to experience the contrary and that's when we need to remind ourselves that we have to do all that we need to in order to stay (or reach) those healthy levels.**

There may be some of you reading this who are battling diseases, aches, pains and ailments - to those people I say that tackling those ailments, aches and pains via a few ways would be great (if you aren't already doing these things). Taking care of ourselves with good mental health practices, good physical health practices while also praying for the best health and visualizing ourselves in the best health are the best and most effective ways to tackle any such problems. God has created us to be whole and healthy but sometimes, we start to experience the contrary and that's when we need to remind ourselves that we have to do all that we need to in order to stay (or reach) those healthy levels.

For instance, I love fast food but I am also mindful that if I keep eating those foods (foods that are high in saturated fats, cholesterol, and processed foods) regularly, I am going to gain weight, I will not have the nutrition I need for a healthy mind and body because processed foods strip the foods of their natural vitamins, and I will be putting myself at-risk for cardiovascular diseases and much more. So, the old adage is true, and the following foods are excellent to ensure optimal health. (Now, I recognize that there are people that have some food allergies and food sensitivities so please consult with your health care provider for exact options that are best for you. Please also check with your health care provider to see if and why some of these foods are not agreeing with you). Here is a list of some really good-for-you foods:

* lean proteins like fish (wild caught is best), chicken (white is lower in calories and fat), lean beef, tofu and tempeh
* water
* herbal teas or teas with caffeine
* fresh fruits and vegetables
* healthy carbohydrates like quinoa, beans and chickpeas
* grains like sunflower seeds, rice, and wheat
* other proteins like eggs or egg whites
* foods low in saturated and trans fats, including low or no cholesterol, salt and sugars

Fueling our bodies is so important and we need to be fair to ourselves: if we don't eat properly, we are simply not going to feel our best and we won't be able to perform at our best. One of the reasons fruits and vegetables are so good for us is because they not only contain a beautiful amount of vitamins and nutrients but they also are water-rich foods which help fuel our bodies.

Now, many people also rely on caffeine and coffee to help fuel them. I myself am one of those people and while I am not a dietitian, naturopath or nutritionist, I can tell you that having a cup or two with a shot or two or three of espresso is generally not going to do anything detrimental to your health and will help you feel alert and "with-it" during times when you need to be especially alert.

Non-Dairy Foods

I have to touch on this point in a chapter that speaks about nutrition because I myself am lactose intolerant and it's a terrible feeling when you are trying to feel good and slim and you instead feel bloated and like you need to run to the bathroom. If you are sensing those things, a trip to the doctor or your healthcare provider would be a good idea but as one who has had to limit dairy for many years, I rely heavily on almond milk, soy milk, non-dairy yogurt, and oat milk. These things are very important because they do allow you to consume the calcium you will need and also don't put that lactose strain on your body. Lactose-free milk is also a great one to use.

Don't Just Jump On the Bandwagon

It is important to be mindful of what we are doing and eating and not just jumping on a trend bandwagon - just because others are avoiding this or that, we don't necessarily have to follow suit. So, do your own research, consult your medical doctor and a nutrition doctor as well, to see what your particular needs are. In other words, people may be avoiding a certain item in foods because they have dietary restrictions but you may not have those same restrictions, so you can still consume those items.

I was speaking to one lady who mentioned to me that she no longer touches gluten. I asked her why. She said that everybody seems to now be avoiding gluten, so why shouldn't she? She also noted that a friend of hers avoided gluten and lost lots of weight. While that reasoning may seem sound, she didn't factor in that her friend could also be doing many other things to achieve the weight loss she was experiencing. It is really important to do what is right for you and to get sound medical and nutritional advice before jumping on the proverbial bandwagon.

Getting Support Of All Kinds

As one who has had to deal with sometimes-crushing news, be it for my health, for my family, for weight loss, etc., support can be so good and so important. Support could mean many different things for many different people and it's so important to give ourselves the best chances for success by arming ourselves with everything possible for best results.

For example, a weight loss company I used provided a few helpful support channels: an app for community messaging, and sharing of pictures, weekly face to face and online support meetings, a number you could call when (at 2 am) you are trying to steer clear of those cookies and more.

The fact is, people need support. We were built by God for community, for support, for fellowship. I think this would go a bit of a way to explaining why social media has exploded over the last few years - we were built to need the support and it caters directly to that. This means that it would be beneficial to you to write out who exists within your support system - who are the people you can turn to for help, support and encouragement when you feel overwhelmed or like you need someone to talk to.

Take a moment right now and use the space provided below to jot down the people you can turn to when you need some help with this. If you feel you would like more people, pray about this and see where God is guiding you. He may be guiding you to include more people who are already in your life who can be of great support to you but maybe you just haven't tapped into that or He may guide you to support groups, etc.

Remember, there is no shame in needing support. Having good and helpful support is so important: people who try to divert your attention away from your health goals and are instead encouraging you to eat that cake or those desserts are not the support you need here.

My list of people who provide me with support:

We all want to feel good and like we're not the only ones going through something. Support allows us to know and to share with others that we are going through "such and such" and allows you to access and connect with others who may be going through the exact same thing or something similar. Either way, it helps us to know that we are not alone in this and that there are others who are also working to accomplish their goals, who are also looking to feel better, who are also trying to be the best version of themselves.

Working Out

Working out is so tremendously important. People who do some form of physical activity in a day report feeling better, feeling lighter, and report overall better health. If taking walks is your thing, do that; if running is your thing, go right ahead. It doesn't always really matter what the physical activity is, what matters is you're doing it and putting your effort into doing it daily or a few times per week. Working out and doing physical exercise is also a great way to keep the blood flowing and circulating through your body, causing increased blood flow to the brain (which helps you think better), allows for delayed onset of wrinkles because your blood is flowing more thoroughly and much more.

At the start of the pandemic, people everywhere were scrambling for a way to work out and to be physically fit, considering gyms and workout facilities were closed. People were looking for all kinds of ways to access fitness machines, take walks, and work out, even in their homes. When I realized that the pandemic was not going to end quickly and that I would need an alternative to the gym I was going to, I went ahead and bought a very simple but functional treadmill. I then had the added task of having to assemble it because no assembly people were taking appointments to come into the home. Anyone who knows me knows that I am not at all great at assembling anything but I realized that it's either do this or have no workout machine. There was also the fact that I had been out walking and running outside (when it was bitterly cold) and got the sniffles more than a couple of times.

Keeping reminders and visual displays are also such an important part of helping ourselves to support ourselves. We can get caught up with the day's busyness and we can make working out and physical health a secondary (if not tertiary or worse) thought and then our body and our mental health suffers as a result. Again, I cover this in much greater detail in my book, Manifest It!

Protein Powders

After a good workout, it can be really helpful to use protein powder in a shake to help replenish your muscles and protein powders can be a good way to accomplish that and can give us a much-needed shot of protein to help us stay and feel full. People often don't get enough protein in their day to begin with, so this can be a good way to help yourself accomplish this.

Yoga, Breathing and Stretching

Yoga is such a wonderful form of exercise, a great way to breathe and to be in sync with your body. The basis of yoga is stretching, controlling one's breathing and training your body to become more fit and more malleable. It is also an excellent intro to simple stretches and to opening up pathways in the body for increased blood flow, causing an overall increase in better health practices. When we breathe deep breaths, we are allowing oxygen to permeate our brains, allowing for greater oxygenated blood to be coursing through our bodies. The great thing about yoga is that it can be done virtually anywhere and with just a simple mat to provide cushioning for your body. It also doesn't have to be a strenuous activity because you can go slowly and take baby steps in your progress. Putting on soothing and calming music would also help to facilitate this and would allow for a more calm mind, allowing you to set behind you current problems or worries you may be having.

The old Cheers song lyrics "taking a break from all your worries sure would help a lot" is so true. When we gain distance from our problems, we begin to look at things differently and we begin to treat our problems differently. We begin to see opportunity when otherwise see strife, unrest, frustration and difficulty. Yoga also helps with this because it can allow for a renewing of our mind.

Taking a Moment

Let's just say that you don't have time to do a full yoga routine that day and you need a moment where you can stop, breathe and re-center to gain calmness and perspective. Staying still (while standing or sitting), closing your eyes and breathing in deeply, praying for the Lord to help you find peace and happiness regardless of the givens of the moment is a tremendously powerful exercise. I have undertaken this exercise myself (I practice what I preach) and have found that a few full breaths of fresh air are fantastic and go a very long way to soothe your worries and nerves. Even if you can't get to a calm space for a few minutes, it is very helpful to pray to the Lord for His help, perspective, wisdom and understanding.

Now, I do want to take a moment and explain that the yoga, praying and breathing I am outlining here is not part of any new age practices. The focus of all the practices I am outlining in this book and in all of my books are practices that focus on Jesus and with help from the Holy Spirit.

16

Focus on Jesus

When we spend time focusing on Jesus, we open ourselves up to the riches and glory that are available in Him, which means all the riches and glory in the world. Jesus has complete dominion over all the world and when we are close enough to Him, patient and we follow His will and guidance, we have access to all the happiness, health, glory, peace and wonder that are available in Him. I have had conversations with those who are Christian but who challenge me when I say that we are supposed to have riches in Christ; that there is nothing wrong with being rich and that when God is our Source, and He has given us the tools to access and to build wealth, there is no harm in using it. In fact, two instances in Scripture come to mind to help me make my point here and after each, I will provide my explanation and breakdown:

Proverbs 21:5 The plans of the diligent lead to profit as surely as haste leads to poverty.

Explanation: First, the diligent plan. If we fail to plan, we will surely plan to fail. If you don't have a plan in mind about how you will do something, it will not go well and you will not experience success. Planning starts with setting your goals and knowing what it is you want to accomplish. Without that, how can you know if you are even on the right track? Secondly, you have to be patient (the opposite of hasty).

God is a God who takes His time but gets it done and done right. Many Christians who have experienced God's goodness will tell you that God works but that He takes His time and He gets something done right. Otherwise, we are making decisions hastily, and we are moving forward in the wrong ways. Moving forward in the wrong ways does mean that you are moving forward in vain - it will not ultimately lead to anything fruitful.

So, when we plan and we are diligent in pursuing those plans (we are organized, we allow ourselves to be led by God, we know that He is guiding each one of our steps) that shows that we are being diligent. Exercise patience while also being diligent and you will reap the benefits. Poverty will be far from you. This is just one of the promises available in Christ.

Matthew 25:14-30 "For it is just like a man about to go on a journey, who called his own slaves and entrusted his possessions to them. To one he gave five talents, to another, two, and to another, one, each according to his own ability; and he went on his journey. Immediately the one who had received the five talents went and traded with them, and gained five more talents. In the same manner the one who had received the two talents gained two more. But he who received the one talent went away, and dug a hole in the ground and hid his master's money. Now after a long time the master of those slaves came and settled accounts with them. The one who had received the five talents came up and brought five more talents, saying, 'Master, you entrusted five talents to me. See, I have gained five more talents.' His master said to him, 'Well done, good and faithful slave You were faithful with a few things, I will put you in charge of many things; enter into the joy of your master.' Also the one who had received the two talents came up and said, 'Master, you entrusted two talents to me. See, I have gained two more talents.' His master said to him, 'Well done, good and faithful slave. You were faithful with a few things, I will put you in charge of many things; enter into the joy of your master.' And the one also who had received the one talent came up and said, 'Master, I knew you to be a hard man, reaping where you did not sow and gathering where you scattered no seed. And I was afraid, and went away and hid your talent in the ground. See, you have what is yours.' But his master answered and said to him, 'You wicked, lazy slave, you knew that I reap where I did not sow and gather where I scattered no seed. 'Then you ought to have put my money in the bank, and on my arrival I would have received my money back with interest. Therefore take away the talent from him, and give it to the one who has the ten talents.' For to everyone who has, more shall be given, and he will have an abundance; but from the one who does not have, even what he does have shall be taken away. Throw out the worthless slave into the outer darkness; in that place there will be weeping and gnashing of teeth."

Explanation: God wants to trust us with all He has (which is everything) but we first have to prove ourselves to Him. We have to show that we will be diligent and faithful in what we do. So, He starts us off with little tests and we have to pass those first, before He gives us more to handle. Doesn't that make good, logical sense? Why would He give us more when we haven't proven ourselves with the little first? Said differently, if He gave us more without first testing us with the little, wouldn't He be setting us up for failure? That is not in God's loving personality.

Further, we need to know Him and understand how He works. We need to understand that He works in great ways which may be different from how we think. We have to get onto His way of thinking; not the other way around.

So, just as in this parable, He entrusts people with little to see what they would do with it and in this parable, the one who did nothing but gave Him back exactly what He had been given initially, had the little taken away from Him and given to one who better managed the resource. This may seem like an unkind thing to do to some people but He is 1) teaching us to be good stewards of wealth and 2) He gives second and third and fourth chances to get it right. It's not like the person in the parable wouldn't have had an opportunity to go at it again and do better. No, God is a God of second and third and fourth chances.

We also see from this parable that God expects good from us and wants good things for us.

Another wonderful thing is that in our conversations with God, we can go to Him and ask Him for His wisdom, to better understand what He wants from us in a given situation. Each situation He puts us in has the potential to make us better, smarter, more quick-on-our-feet and to make more strategic decisions. It is the wise person indeed who can see this and use it to their advantage.

The same self-proclaimed atheist I referred to earlier in the book took me up on my suggestion to read Proverbs. I invited her to read it and to let me know what she understood from it, and invited her to discuss it with me following her read. I do not exaggerate when I say that she was not yet finished the book of Proverbs when she said she could feel the wisdom and the intelligence from this book. She was calling the book of God one of the wisest books she had ever read. I was so pleased to hear that because many who say that they don't believe in God won't even open themselves up to reading His word, let alone express how wise it is.

God's Ways Are Not Our Ways

This is a very important point: In all your ways acknowledge Him. God has ways that we cannot understand. He is not limited to the laws of physics, or to any other laws. He is limited by nothing. As such, when we don't see a way around things, please understand that He has a way and He will use it to benefit you, His child. That's just one reason why we must turn to Him and this is a very important point I wish to cover in this chapter that is all about focusing our eyes and the eyes of our heart on Jesus.

When we are stuck in a problem, we often do not see a way out. In fact, we may be downright panicked and when that happens (I don't care who you are or how old you are, the same rule applies), we stop thinking strategically. The best thing to do is to calm down and let God do what He needs to do. Let God take control of the situation, dire as it may seem. I also cover this concept in my illustrated book, Give it to God, but will be explaining more thoroughly in this book.

When you focus your eyes on Jesus and you let Him take control, you will see wonderful things move in the right direction - and that means the direction that will cause you to arrive at a great solution. It is for that reason that we need to pray, we need to stop and listen also to what He is communicating to us and that we need to obey Him. For example, if He is leading you to stay away from a certain person, He has a very good reason and you would be wise to listen and to obey. He knows that person and their heart in a way that you do not. He knows that person's heart and intentions in a way that you never can. And He will not ask you to stay away from a person when they are good for you. I used to read subway posters that detailed Scripture, and read "Do not lean on your own understanding" and that is so true.

My experience has shown again and again that when I lean on my own understanding, I miss lots of important information, I can misread things and I can misunderstand things. I'll give you a for-instance: I met someone through work that I thought was the best. He was handsome, seemed sweet, kind and totally knowledgeable...the whole package. He was always well-dressed, and while he kept to himself, I sensed that he had a wisdom beyond his years.

Boy was I wrong!

God must have whispered to me so many times to stay away, stay away, stay away. I stupidly leaned on my own understanding and got close to him. I was friendly with him, tried to enjoy good conversation, and made efforts to invite him out and include him, not to mention offered to help with any resources he may need. Basically, I was as friendly as can be. What I got in return and experienced quickly was a very selfish, self-centered man who could not care less about anything else or anyone else. I even had a fellow co-worker share that her experience with him was also not positive and that he was acting like a total jerk. I persisted. I kept inviting him out, being kind, and believing the best of him. Well, I ended up realizing that my efforts were totally in-vain and that there was no point in putting time and energy into this man. I learned the hard way how unkind, rude and frankly, deceitful he had been.

On the Flip Side

Just as the sub-heading goes, I also have a flip-side to tell you about. I met someone that I wasn't very impressed with from the beginning. He seemed selfish and unkind, very full of himself. When I prayed to the Lord about it, He pointed out that the outer shell of this person was not accurate and that he was actually a very kind and good soul. I was floored. I was convinced that this person was a jerk. Regardless, because of circumstances, I started getting to know him and spending time with him. As the layers peeled back, I began to notice that there was an incredible sweetness, kindness and goodness to him, something I never would have seen had I stuck to my earlier thoughts and just walked away.

That's just one of the huge benefits of focusing on Jesus and consulting with the Holy Spirit : every time we are wondering about something and we need to know what's at the heart of the situation, what this person is really like or what they are really like, we get to know the truth about a person and hear about their truth directly from the One who created them. We get to understand that God knows exactly what is at heart with each person and in each situation. There is more than enough pain and suffering in this world so when He is leading you away from something or someone, we would be wise to listen and to obey, knowing full well and being assured that He is saying it for our benefit. In sum, it's really an amazing thing when the truth is revealed to us, whether it lines up with what we thought or not.

Someone reading this could be thinking: *"Well that's great for you, Christine, but how am I supposed to know if I'm being led or not?"* Friend, if you are asking the Holy Spirit, you are being led because everyone who seeks, finds and everyone who asks will receive. The Holy Spirit does not just like me better or another Christian better. No, He will answer your questions and provide you with truth regardless of where you are in your Christian walk. All you have to do is pay attention and obey.

Now, what happens if you asked, and received but you didn't obey (and it did or did not blow up in your face)? Is all lost? Definitely not. That's why we repent for being disobedient or for our unbelief and we move forward to better. And when I say better, I mean a more solid relationship with God, one where we know Him a little better now and so when He is advising us of something, we actually listen and we actually obey. This is what building our faith is all about and it's an important step of the process. I would be a liar if I said that I didn't have to repent a few times for my unbelief and/or for disobedience. But each time I did, I was given an opportunity to turn things around and end up with, ultimately, a more solid relationship with God. Remember, He knew from the beginning that we would mess up (and more than once) - that's why we have repentance and forgiveness and moving forward.

17

Strive for More, Better, Higher

I could not mean this more: raise your standards, go for higher, go for better.

Now, there is nothing wrong with starting at the "bottom" and paying your dues. Certainly not. There is something to be admired in a person who does that. This chapter is about starting there and becoming such a diligent, caring, giving worker that your employer sees that and wants to promote you because you work so hard and you are dedicated to what you are doing.

As a child of God, created by Him, you are the son or daughter of the King of Kings. This means that you have greatness in you (every single one of you). You have talents, skills and abilities that are unique to you and that are part of what make you so amazing. It could be culinary skills, painting or sculpting, teaching, engineering, being a great doctor of medicine, a great and gifted actor, comedian or producer and director, it could be being an amazing homemaker and making your home an amazing place for your husband and or wife and kids, it could be being a great vet who lovingly looks after the needs of little and big animals, a botanist or horticulturalist, a great fashion designer or a tech guru. The list is endless because there are so many great courses of work (some that I mentioned are unpaid but still invaluable) and skills and talents required by each and they all have certainly at least one thing in common: the ability to be great, outstanding and get better and better as you go.

Some people can get comfortable and complacent, not thinking about or wanting to move up, and therefore they don't put their best into what they do; they get to work late, they don't put in their best work while they are there, they are not an effective team player, they don't follow instructions carefully or really listen, they are dragging the team down through one way or another....the list can go on. If this is you, you are not putting your best into what you do. It takes a strong person to self-reflect and to realize that they haven't put their best into what they are doing and then to change course and begin to put in their best into what they are doing. Making this change takes presence of mind and a renewed dedication that you are doing this because it is what God has called you to do and therefore you want to do it well.

I know a very gifted chef who scored himself a position (it was not a high chef position but nonetheless) in a very swanky, upscale restaurant in Las Vegas. He had baked and cooked in front of me before so I could see just how good he was. He was a very gifted chef. The problem was that he didn't put his heart and soul into it. He would complain all the time about the work conditions, and about how unfair it was that he wasn't higher up already (he had just started the position). He went through his days feeling unhappy and as a result, was not putting his best into his work, not giving it his all. He did, in fact, get a promotion and was very happy about it but still was not happy that he wasn't further up and the lead chef in the kitchen. These feelings continued to seep into his work and years later, while he did get promoted over the years because he was very good at his work and had raw talent, his lack of appreciation for where he was and his skills kept plaguing him. It is really unfortunate because years later, he talked to me about his lousy attitude when things really did get hard in another workplace and spoke to me about having wished he was more thankful for the good breaks and good beginning he did get.

Sometimes, friends and readers, it isn't about your position. You will move on from that position and hopefully you will be able to look back and say that you did your best and you put your all into this position so that when you do get promoted, you will know you deserved that promotion. One of the most wonderful things about working at something God has called you to do is to know that when the going gets tough, you can rely on Him to make things better and you can rely on Him to promote you, even when those around you won't. You are working for Him and as long as you maintain a positive attitude, as long as you keep honoring Him, He will move you forward because that's God honoring you back.

Continuing to Hone Your Skills

It is so important to continue to hone your skills and to continue to get better. There are constantly new ways and new developments coming up and we need to make sure that we are keeping our skills sharp and up-to-date. This will require continually reading, learning, dedicating yourself to continuing to get better and it will necessarily require you to ask questions and to stretch yourself.

I am reminded of my dad who worked as a dentist all his life, having come to Canada with only his mother and two siblings, and with so little in their pockets that they were all living in a one-bedroom apartment in a not-great area of Toronto. My dad spoke Armenian and Arabic, without a word of English. He was scared (the whole family was) and he was the oldest, so he knew that a tremendous load of responsibility was on him whether he liked it or not. He knew he had to rise to the occasion, get a job, find himself a career that would pay well enough to support his family and work hard and maintain a positive attitude. Thankfully, my dad always always always kept a positive, "can-do" attitude. He always met challenges head-on, such as when he would read his Science books (written in English when he didn't speak English) so he would write the word in Arabic on top of the English word, until he learned English fluently enough that he was able to stop doing that. He also worked his way through university, ensuring that his tuition was paid, the rent was paid, and that his siblings (including a baby sister) were properly cared for and his mother (his father had passed away) who didn't speak a word of English and couldn't work due to ailments, was able to put food on the table each evening.

One of the many things I admire about my dad is his "can-do" attitude throughout his life. He has always been such a good, kind, caring provider, even providing when he knew it was stretching him big time! And that's one of the best gifts and lessons we can pass on to our kids: work hard and diligently and with a very positive attitude because you are working for God, not for man. You keep a good attitude and say your prayers and do your best and it is God who will promote you, not man.

Before retiring, my dad used to always read up on new dental tricks and ways, and used to attend conventions touting the latest technologies and the latest procedures. This was always important to him because even though many of his patients were a bit more senior, he wanted to give them the best service and use the latest products for the best service possible. That was and is the kind of man my dad is and a great lesson he passed on to us, his kids.

Who Are You Close To?

I ask this question because it's always a good idea to maintain good relationships and to spend time with people who know more and know better than you, people who can show you how to strive for better and who put their best into what they do. The people you surround yourself with are so important to your development and your progress because when we are around people who don't constantly strive for better, for more, for greater results, we become very complacent and we become stagnant.

I caution you when I say this, though, because there are some people who may give the impression of being cutting edge and "with-it" but are just showing off. To illustrate, I had a friend years ago who showed up in gorgeous cars, lived in the swankiest neighborhood, had investment properties here and there, would get her hair done once per week, dressed to the nines, was always talking about the next million dollar deal, etc. I admit that at the time, I was green with envy. I thought she had everything and I was dying to know more, dying to be part of that world, to be included. Well, I discovered that there was a nice and lovely illusion there - to put it mildly. I was not willing to do the underhanded things she was doing to get those material goods. I will never forget when she began talking to me about her spiritual lifestyle and encouraged me to do the same and admittedly, I dabbled in it. I realized years later how my envy and misconception of her life led me to believe that she had so much more than me and how I wasn't doing things correctly or correctly enough. Today, I am so very grateful that I don't follow those practices and that my faith and my self-worth is firmly rooted in Christ.

In sum, keeping our eyes on Jesus and allowing the Holy Spirit to guide you is the best guidance you can get because all the riches, the promotions, the good breaks we will ever need are found in Him.

To close this chapter, I want to remind you and encourage you, dear reader, to ask God to speak to your heart and to see how He suggests you improve, how He suggests you move forward and to better yourself, and how He guides you to do all of those things. Use that trusty journal you started and record what He says to you and how He guides you. You will be able to look back on these notes months or years from now and know with satisfaction that you followed Him to a more lucrative life and to a more successful life!

18
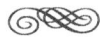

Remember Who You Are In Christ On Those Hard Days

I want to make this clear: nobody but nobody said this was going to be easy. Success. Nobody said success was going to be easy and that's unfortunately something we all have to contend with.

We all have those difficult days. We all have those days where the challenges seem and feel insurmountable and where things are just not working the way that we want them to. A co-worker got the promotion, the business deal fell through, our worker quit when we needed them the most, our boss does not see us as the leader that we see ourselves, among other things. Those days do happen and it takes a lot of strength of character and it takes a lot of reminding ourselves why we are doing what we are doing to keep going on those days in particular. As children of God, we have the ability and we have at our disposal God's protection and the way that can be opened through Him and Him alone. This means that the going will get tough and that obstacles will abound in front of us but He is going to remove or supersede or overrule those obstacles if it is His will and in His timing.

I have definitely come to realize that one of the ways that you know that something is God's will is if He makes the way for it to happen.

If you ask Him in the midst of the difficulties to open the way for the miracle to happen , He will always respond and guide you. He may say that this difficulty is for a finite time and that He will get you out of it, He may guide you to learn from it, or He may guide how you can get yourself out of it with His help.

One such instance of this that I am reminded of most recently is when I was trying to register my very first production for a media series that I wanted to put together. I knew that this was something that God was calling me to do and besides the obstacles of seemingly-insurmountable amounts of paperwork that at first glance seemed incredibly daunting and with no help or support available to me, I realized that I had to navigate these unchartered waters with only the promptings of the Holy Spirit. My initially submitted paperwork was completely ignored by the organization that was supposed to give their stamp of approval and they were the only ones who could provide this stamp of approval. Upon further prayer, I was asking the Lord if this is really the way that He wants me to go and the answer kept coming back as a "yes". So I called the organization and while the lady responsible came across as one of the most unpleasant people I have ever had the misfortune of dealing with, and who told me in no uncertain terms, actually accused me of things that I was just not guilty of and belittled my production completely. When I clarified my intentions and stood up for myself and pointed out that she didn't even know me and that she was accusing me of things and then made a silent prayer in my head that if this is what He wanted, that He was going to have to open the door. Not five minutes later she apologized to me for her rudeness and offered to process the paperwork right away, providing me with the necessary wording to expedite things. The following day I got my approvals for the project and that is now part of history because the project did get approved and got made. Getting the project made was no easy feat - it was difficult, cumbersome, time-consuming, and I had no human outside help. The Lord does not promise us that we will not have difficulties but He does promise us that He will be with us in those difficulties.

I sometimes then think about all those people in the world who are experiencing problems and difficulties, whether it's in one field or another, whether it's in their personal lives or in their career lives and how they may be wondering to themselves if this endeavor is God's will for their lives. Without having an active, living, and vibrant relationship with Him, we have no way of actually knowing that. I am reminded of a lady that I used to know who had been married for a little while and was looking to have her first child. They were experiencing some difficulties and I had asked her if she had prayed about the situation. She said that she had not but that it is very possible that this was not God's will for her life. At that point in time, I already had the relationship of hearing from the Lord the way that I do and I was able to tell her that I believe that it is God's will for her to have a child and that she should use the following strategies to help make it happen and help make conception a reality. When I told her about this, she became very upset with me. It has been several years since that event happened and even though this person is not in my life, I still go back and reflect on whether I should have done something differently. I did reaffirm through much reflection and prayer that unfortunately, her unbelief was the barrier that was in the way. She had mentioned that there was no biological and scientific reason for which she could not get pregnant and I definitely sense that it was her lack of faith and lack of belief that was causing this.

When the Lord is giving us His go-ahead and green light to proceed with something despite the difficulties that are in front of us, we need to move forward. It is fine to take a momentary step back and pray for His strength because we are not supposed to do these things in our own strengths and abilities. If I could say to this lady now that it is years later and who is still childless, I would encourage her to have more faith and to get out of her own way.

This is part of the beauty of having our identity in Christ: we have a loving, caring, ever-present supernatural God who is in our corner, just like He was in David's corner, Moses' corner, Mary's corner, Abraham's corner, and many more in Scripture. **He is still the God of miracles and He is still the God who does much good, we just need to rely on Him and His strength.**

We Are Sheep

This is why we are called sheep. Sheep, without their shepherd, would be totally lost and very much at the dangerous hands of the big bad wolf. When we don't stay close to the Shepherd (God), we put ourselves in a very vulnerable position and we open ourselves up to the whims and whiles of the enemy. We open ourselves up to constant bombardment, harassment and we are totally subject to our own limited and solely human way of seeing things.

I ask the question, therefore: why would we not rather choose to be close to the Shepherd, who is there to love us, to care for us, is responsible for us and protects us? I don't think too many would disagree that there are many dangerous people, events and circumstances in our world, for both adults and for children. Why would we think we would do better without the Shepherd's help? Why would we not teach our children to rely on God because as much as even the most loving of parents can be, we cannot be there 100% of the time to help our children. We have to turn over their wellness and well-being to God, Who is there, and able to watch over our children in a way that is supernatural.

Personally, I know that I would have been able to excel much more and much earlier in life had I known the goodness and power that was available to me in Christ. It would have been very helpful if I had been taught that I can (and am supposed to) have my own relationship with Christ and what that looks like and how that actually comes to happen in real life terms. Raised a Christian, I did not know this until I was well into my thirties, at which point it took a good friend at least a couple of years to pray for me to see the proverbial light.

It is very gratifying every time a friend, family member or a person tells me that my books are helping their child or children or themselves. One friend one evening sent me a screenshot of her purchase of my books and how her daughters were now getting into the habit of praying to Jesus. She even sent me a picture of her older daughter in the closet, on her knees, praying with her eyes closed. My heart soared and I melted all at the same time. For this young and precious little girl to have discovered the benefit of prayer and for her to have turned to the Lord in prayer (whether it was her first prayer or she was a veteran at praying), she was given the greatest gift of all: that of faith. She was able to start her relationship with Christ at a young age and to rely on truth that is available in Him and Him only.

Churches

It always amazes me when people refer to a negative experience with a clergy member and translate that to "God doesn't care", "God is not good", "God is not for me". I have had many unfortunate encounters with clergy members and I have discovered one thing: they are NOT God. They are human beings and they will make mistakes. It was never a member of the clergy who taught me that I can have that living and vibrant relationship with Christ and definitely none of them taught me how to do that. That is something I learned from watching my friend, from asking my God-father questions, from listening to sermons from anointed pastors and preachers like Joyce Meyer, Joel Osteen, Jurgen Matthesius, Brett McBride, Charles Stanley and many more. I learned all about how God works and by seeing and experiencing first-hand the results obedience brings and seeing first-hand the results disobedience brings. I am very grateful for the courses in my Doctoral program which provided resource after resource about this vibrant relationship and how paper after paper was not just about who God is in theory but in application. I had countless lessons where I had to state something as it was pre-prayer and pre-action, record my prayer and then give it some time to see what happens post-prayer.

Having said all of this, would I like for the Church to be a more anointed place, a place where people can discover the live and vibrant relationship that exists in Christ? Absolutely. The Church is Christ's love and needs to be that place where people can go to feel all of the following:

- Loved
- Seen
- Heard
- Accepted
- Helped
- Brought into active relationship with Christ

The Church is supposed to be a place where all people feel loved and welcome, but it still needs to be a place where the values of God are upheld, respected and practiced. I have seen few Churches where confession is a regular practice, where deliverance is done openly and not in hiding, where a clergy member might actually turn a couple away because it is not God's will for them to be united, and more. Churches have a tremendous responsibility to uphold the right and correct will of God, but it is only with people knowing God, the Word and His personality that they will accept these as truth and will adhere to them. I know that for me, it took me time to really understand, internalize and respect God and then love and respect His ways. Without this level of closeness and love, it was harder for me to really be obedient and to understand that when He says something, He means it.

> **I know that for me, it took me time to really understand, internalize and respect God and then love and respect His ways.**

You Will Experience Setbacks

Everyone does.

On the road to success, personal or professional or both, you will experience setbacks. Setbacks can be major or they can be minor but they will come your way. The question then becomes: how do we defeat and overcome those hurdles?

It's very simple. Ask God.

God knows exactly what to do, He knew this setback was coming (it was not and is not) a surprise to Him. So, when I say ask God, this is the process I use:

1. Get into a comfortable, quiet place where you can really be at one with your thoughts.
2. Pray and thank the Lord for your blessings and let Him know about your feelings about this setback. Talk to Him about all parts of it as much as you like.
3. Ask for His help - ask Him what He would have you do to help you through this. Ask Him not only what to do but when to do it and tell Him that you are coming to Him and counting on Him for His help. Ask Him to speak to you clearly and directly to your heart.
4. Stop and listen. You may get words pop into your mind. You may get an idea. You may get a feeling about something. Either way, the Holy Spirit is going to answer you and is going to help you.
5. Ask for confirmation that this is from Him if you need it and to keep out of your mind all other voices or influences.

It May Not Make Total Sense To You

Something that I think is rather important to mention here is that the response you get may not make a lot of sense to you. It may suggest and guide you to do something that you normally wouldn't do and it may guide you to take an action that would seem out of character for you. Just go with it. We don't always have to understand what we're being guided to do, but we need to do it if we want to see those improvements.

I recall a time when I was asked to do something completely outside of my understanding. It didn't make any sense why I was guided to do that and it was something that was very out of character for me. Somewhat begrudgingly, I did it anyway. The results were not what I could have expected in any way...they were much better.

Go To God First

People often make the mistake of first going to a family, friend or someone else to get help and perspective on their problems. With all due respect to my reader, this is not really correct. God does often work through people, yes, but we have to go to God first for His take. We have to clue Him in to what's going on - not because He doesn't already know, but because He wants to be actively involved in your life and wants to help you through things. If you use the steps I just outlined, you can be sure that He will answer you, He will help you, He will guide you, He will support you. Said differently, He longs for you to come to Him, to ask Him, to help you, so when you engage in these steps, you are doing just that. Trust me when I say that He will certainly answer you.

Now, the answer may take some time to come and, or it may take time to implement. This does not mean that God is saying "No, I won't help you."

Takes Time to Implement?

What do I mean by this? I mean that it may take some time to implement and to come out with a good resolution to your problem. It may take time for things to move into the direction of being resolved. Problems normally do take some time to be resolved, and this is no different. Having said that, if you ask God to expedite the process, He may do that but it still ultimately takes some time.

I'll give you the example of a nice lady I had the great fortune of coming across. She was very sweet and she had a daughter who was adopted. She had been up-front with the girl that she was adopted and they talked things out. The daughter frankly adored her adopted mom (the nice lady I knew) but things came to a head when her biological mother (who had been in and out of prison for years) came into her life and wanted to be a part of her life again. She had not yet finished her prison term and was experiencing problems with drugs and alcohol abuse. She was not interested in getting help for these issues but she still wanted an active relationship with her biological daughter. The nice lady wasn't sure what to do because she was afraid of the effects this would have on her adopted daughter. She became alarmed when she found a package of cigarettes in her room. So, I advised the nice lady to pray and to seek God's face in this very difficult situation. God guided her to spend time with her adopted daughter, reminding her of the good values she had instilled in her and asking her to spend time with her doing their usual low-key but cherished activities: reading, attending music concerts, shopping for food and clothes, making healthy food and desserts together and watching comedy shows together. It took months and months for real changes to be seen in both of their lives but ultimately, it created a much deeper bond between the nice lady and the adopted daughter, and eventually, the biological mother chose to get help and seek treatment in a facility, opening the door to a possible eventual reconciliation and relationship with her daughter.

This happy resolution took many months and much faith on the part of the nice lady but it happened and it was very good.

Another example I'd like to share with you because it is a heartwarming story is that of a young woman who had low self esteem and she was lured into the human trafficking industry. Her parents were devoted Christians who attended the same Church as I did and were kind, loving people who were desperately praying to have their daughter back and that she would be healed from the mental, physical and emotional trauma that obviously would come from being a victim of human trafficking. One day, this young lady (who was now free from her captives) and her loving parents got up onto the large stage at the Church and presented their daughter's story. The parents said that it had taken years of prayer and hard work to get their daughter to be released but that she eventually was and now it was time to work on the lengthy healing process that would be required.

You see, God's work is not little; there are many things each and every praying person (and even non-praying persons) require but we have to be patient and understand that God is working. He is working even when we don't see Him working. One way that I like to keep this in mind (especially during those times where I am getting impatient and it seems like nothing is working) is to look at the clouds in the sky moving. This helps me in a few ways:

1. God is up there and He is working….He is not a liar that I should think that He is not telling me the truth when He says that He never stops working.
2. I didn't ask the clouds to move…they just do. As such, imagine how much more God will move because we have asked Him to.
3. In Scripture, it says that God neither sleeps nor slumbers. I have to believe that He is up, working on the things that I have brought to His feet.
4. I look back to previous answered prayers as my evidence that if

He did it once, He will do it again. I can also (we all can) look at the answered prayers of others and see how God helped them and that of course, He will help us too.

Try It For Yourself

I never tell anyone I minister to to just take my word for it. Never. I don't think that's really fair. What I do is to tell them of my experiences and invite them to pray about it and have their own experiences with God. Pray for yourself, ask for yourself, inquire for yourself, test Scripture for yourself and see how He responds. God promises us in Scripture that nobody who comes to Him will be turned away and that everyone who repents will be forgiven. This seems like a pretty solid promise to me. So I say, try it for yourself and see what the response is. I do invite people who are looking for help on this to reach out to me via my website's contact form. I had help going through this process and so I only find it right and fair to provide some help and some coaching for others. Please visit drchristinetopjian.com for those details and to reach out.

I also say to check out community forums and Church groups. It is so helpful to have those community resources there, allowing you to see the faith promises and testimonials of others, and having an opportunity to share your own stories. Hearing some of what others go through is so important because it helps us put things into perspective and it helps fuel our own faith. One of my favorite and most heart-warming things to experience is when I see the prayer requests of others on different apps and different websites. I see everything from "Please help my kid find their way" to "Our business is in trouble" to "Please read my heart, Lord, and help us". I love seeing these because I get to experience others coming to Jesus for help and relying on His promises, His character and His goodness to help them through everything.

I always want to encourage my readers to reach out to community support groups, whether face to face in a Bible-based Church or online, these are always such good things to do and such wonderful ways to connect with others. You never know who God puts in your path to help you or how you can help them. These can be a great source of comfort when you are dealing with setbacks and you need others to provide some support and some perspective. It can also be a great source of providing a testimonial for how Jesus helps and helped (present tense and past tense) someone through a difficulty or a setback and gives you an oomf of energy to continue on to your path.

Helping People Through Their Setbacks

I went to a Church prayer meeting one time and while I sensed that God wanted me to go there, I didn't sense that He intended for me to stay there that night. I was totally confused and perplexed. "Go there but don't stay there??? Ok, Lord," I said with a sigh. "As you wish, Lord. Show me what you would like me to do", I said.

I got to the meeting and they were going to start in a matter of a few minutes. I got seated at a table and felt quite comfortable. It turns out that they were all reading and using a workbook I didn't yet have (or know about) so I purchased it for a nominal fee. As I got the booklet and workbook in my hand, I sensed something was about to happen. It did. There was a lady standing at the purchase counter next to me and she was talking about how she wanted to buy the book and workbook but she didn't have enough money. The saleslady didn't know what to do because she was clearly not authorized to let her have the book and workbook free of charge. Just then, I felt in my spirit, "Give her your paid copies and go home. I have other things for you to do tonight." I promptly offered the lady standing next to me my book and workbook and told her it was the Lord's will for her to have my copies and then I politely excused myself from the meeting that had still not yet started. The girl I gave the book and workbook to was floored and just gasped when the book and workbook were transferred into her hand, free of charge. I don't know really how my gesture of obedience affected this girl and I hope she got a lot out of the meeting but it felt nice doing this and I was grateful to have been able to.

My last example of helping someone through a setback is this next example I will provide: a lady I worked with has a husband who is a bit older and was going to get brain surgery shortly. I had spoken to this lady a handful of times and felt connected to her, like she is a kindred spirit. She opened up to me about her husband's surgery and admitted that she was very scared but didn't know how to pray, so when I offered to help her and her family by praying for her husband, she jumped at the offer. A friend of mine and I did pray for her husband and her family and we also prayed that this might open up the lady to a relationship with Jesus. Her husband had the surgery and it went amazingly well, even better than they had hoped for. She did thank me profusely for mine and my friend's help in praying and I can only hope that in some small way, this may have opened the door to her beginning a relationship with Christ.

In sum, readers, setbacks will happen on our route to whatever definition of success you would like to use, but there are many ways to help us through these, not the least of which is Jesus Himself! Rely on Him - He wants you to!

19

Congratulations, You!

I really want to take a moment at this point in the book to say congratulations to you. First, for continuing to read and for having gotten this far in the book. And secondly, to remind you that it's ok (in fact, more than ok) to give yourself that pat on the back and to congratulate yourself for your great work, whatever that great work is. Celebrate the little wins along the way.

Finished a book? Congratulate yourself.
Did your first prayer? Congratulate yourself.
Helped someone today? Congratulate yourself.
Made a nutritious meal for you and your family? Congratulate yourself.
Worked out today? Give yourself a pat on the back.
Did a good job at your job today? Give yourself that pat on the back.
Did that 30 minute walk? Give yourself a nice treat to commend yourself.

Readers, if we don't take time to congratulate ourselves for the little wins, we are missing out on a huge part of the happy-making equation. **Yes, the happy-making equation.** There are more than enough hardships in this world, so when you engage the happy-making equation, you are finding moments and ways to innovatively and in a fun way, celebrate the little good things that you do. Remember that it takes strength, effort, dedication, love, energy, good will and so much more to wear all the hats that we wear.

Here are just some of the many hats we wear. Take a moment and either with a highlighter or a pen or pencil, use the list of items below to remind yourself of the hats you currently wear, will be wearing either soon or hopefully soon or have worn. Even if you wore the hat temporarily, it still counts, use it.

Here is the list and the spaces provided below are for the hats you think of that you'd like to jot down for either hats you have worn that I have not included here (the list is not exhaustive) or for hats you would like to wear in the future:

Caregiver   Parent   Sibling   Auntie   Uncle

Homemaker   Friend   Cousin   Problem-Solver

Confidant(e)   Church-goer   Best friend   Gardener

Teacher   Helper   Patron   Artistic Person

Career Person   Mortgage Payer   Rent Payer   Car Driver

Bike Rider   Musician   Scientist   Homesitter

Praying Person   Step-Parent   Grandparent

Adoptive Parent   Working Out Person   Handyman or Handywoman

_____
_____
_____
_____   _____
_____   _____
_____   _____
_____   _____
_____   _____
           _____
           _____

Why did I suggest this activity? Because it goes to show you how many things you do in a day, in an hour, in a minute that matter so much for your own health and well-being and for (or to) others. For instance, if you are a step-parent, you could very well mean the world to your stepson or stepdaughter - they could look up to you in a way that you may not really yet be aware of and that's something to congratulate yourself for. You could also be the one that pays the mortgage for your family and that's a huge accomplishment and responsibility that needs to be honored and respected and celebrated because your whole family is relying on you to do that, and in order to do that, you will need to have some sort of work and some sort of income, so good on you!

Some people reading this may be thinking *"Well, Christine, that's not really a big deal."* Wrong. I'm here to tell you that it is a big deal and you should be so proud of yourself for doing it. I haven't even yet mentioned the impact that your responsibilities and good works do for those around you, who may very well be observing and watching what you do and are super impressed that you are able to uphold those tasks and duties, each and every time it comes around.

You may choose to congratulate yourself and celebrate a little accomplishment by buying yourself a little something special, and that's great. For example, a lady I know was going through a very difficult pregnancy and had to make many trips to the hospital, and I mean many. It was starting to get her really down and so I suggested that each time she make a trip to the hospital, to do something nice for herself. For her, that meant buying herself some rich, scented soaps for her home's powder room. For me, it would be to buy a custom-made coffee for myself. For another guy I knew who was going through a very difficult divorce and whose wife was basically taking him to the cleaners, each successful time he battled in court, he allowed himself to go to the park and swing on the swings for a while, because this reminded him of happier and simpler times.

So, here are some nice things you can do for yourself. Pick one or many. Enjoy yourself with this exercise. After all, this is your opportunity to reward yourself for having done GOOD!

- Buy yourself flowers
- Buy yourself an action figure
- Get yourself tickets to a sports game or event
- Get yourself something cool gadget-wise
- Buy yourself a designer cup of joe or cup of coffee, made just the way you like
- Have a nice glass of wine or beer
- Take a walk in nature
- Look up and take a good, long look at the stars
- Start a warm fuzzies file
- Hug your pet
- Turn off your phone
- Stretch and do some yoga
- Write your gratitude out
- Get some delicious and healthy food you would love
- Bake or cook something for someone and deliver it to them

- Take a power nap
- Plant something
- Write (by hand) the angriest letter you can to a person who is causing you the most stress. Take a deep breath. Throw it away.
- Spend time in natural sunlight
- Watch a movie
- Take a bubble bath
- Put on some perfume or cologne
- Play with your kids
- Go for a long drive
- Address home improvements that need to be made
- Give someone you know and love a hug
- Decide to read only good and happy news
- Unfollow ten social media accounts that don't bring you joy
- Sign up for a class you'd like to take
- Write that poem or short story or those poems or short stories you've been meaning to
- Try a new recipe
- Drink more water
- Prioritize a good wind-down routine
- Forgive yourself. Give yourself a hug
- Add "Time to laugh" in your calendar
- Take a Flintstones vitamin
- Write down a list of 10 things you love about yourself

Of course, reader, there are many more to add to this list and if this list does not have what you would like, I encourage you to add to it with the things that are meaningful to you. This exercise is meant to be a reward for you and something that you use that will make you feel good after all you take on.

Some people may think that the things they do are just "normal, everyday things." Friend, I'd like to tell you that that's not always the case. Not everyone does the great work you do and puts in the time, energy and effort to do that thing like you do. Not everyone is a great and reliable volunteer at Church and does all they can to make fellow patrons feel welcomed. Not everyone puts their all into their work and goes above and beyond, putting in extra hours and doing their best to make the company successful and profitable. Not everyone takes time to cherish their spouse or their partner to make them feel extra special. We all have things that we do and we think that they are "normal things" that "everyone just does", but that is not the case. Not everyone does those things so you should reward yourself for doing them.God is watching and seeing your dedication, your good works, your efforts and He is another One who will reward you, over and above your own self-rewards.

Those Who Try To Bring You Down

In a chapter on congratulating yourself for a job well done, we have to address those who will (or do) (try to) bring you down. In our society, there are people who try to bring others down because they may be jealous, they may feel threatened, or they just may not like you and so they don't want to support you and some want to outright tear you down. Never mind those people and you keep doing your thing. You keep being the best exactly where God has placed you and you will see things change, and improve. You will see God vindicate you for the wrongs these people have committed. He knew the unfair treatment would be coming and He knew that people would be jealous of you and not wish you well. You cannot let that hinder you. You keep doing what you know you are supposed to be doing and let God deal with handling them with justice.

A lady I know named Nada was going to work each day, doing her best, putting her all into her job. She was kind, respectful, on-time (and usually early) to work, she did her job and she did it well. She was always smiling, in the face of tremendous difficulties in her life. When a job opened up in the customer service department that required a bilingual customer service person, she suggested the job to me and I put in my application. I got the job and was so grateful to her. We used to sit together and have lunch, and she used to talk to me about why she loved her job at the company as a scientist, how fulfilled she felt with what she was doing each day, and how hard she worked for the company. Unfortunately, her immediate boss did not appreciate her or note the good works she was doing. He would belittle her efforts, he would say mean and hurtful things, he would misjudge her on all fronts. She had gotten used to it but at the same time, the mean and hurtful things he would say stayed with her, but she kept being her best, putting her all into her work, trying to tune out what he would say to her. The time came when that person was eventually let go from the company and the new boss could see her hard work, her dedication and her efforts and he decided to promote her.

What am I saying? God sees all the justices and injustices and He will promote you and raise you at the perfect time.

Incidentally, I did mention to Nada that she should take some time for herself each week to thank herself for her wonderful work and she should do something kind and good for herself. She decided to take me up on that and each week, she did one thing that made her feel good. I believe she is still doing that to this day, as I write this.

At one of Jane's jobs, she had some workers who clearly did not like her. They hid their disdain for her very poorly and definitely thought she was not a winner. I remember one morning, Jane was telling me how she got in to work late because there had been a terrible blizzard and snowstorm. Her car wouldn't get out of the driveway and she took the bus to get to work that day, having to trudge through the snow to get to work. Once there, Jane's boss thanked her very kindly for coming in and for braving the blizzard, but when she got to her work space, one of the ladies who also worked there made a very snide comment against her. I reminded Jane that she should not spend time and energy on people like that and that the work she was doing was for the Lord.

So, as they do for us all, naysayers will come, people who enjoy (or seem to enjoy) making our lives difficult will come, they will say things and do things that are uncalled for, unprofessional and unkind but we cannot let them get the best of us. We have to let the offense go and pay no mind. Let God pay them back for what they have said and done.

What Is a Little Win?

What is a little win? A little win is a step in the right direction toward where you want to be and where you are called to be. It is a step toward success in your goals. Each of the following are little wins that have either happened to me, a friend of mine, a family member or to someone I have in some way ministered to. After this list, I will be asking you to think about it and jot down some little wins you have experienced on your road to success. See, each one of these little wins must be celebrated because success, real success, takes time so this is your way of motivating yourself to continue on the road to the fulfillment of your goals and in reminding yourself that *"Yes, I am on the right track and despite the challenges, I am slowly but surely making my way through."*

Examples of little wins:

- I am making really good headway in my new course
- We are not pregnant yet but we had our first IVF session and so we are on the right track
- I met someone special and was totally myself. I'm excited to see where this goes.
- I successfully completed & submitted my essay applications for my university applications

- I aced my presentation at work today
- I delivered a great lesson for my students today and I think they really got it
- I wrote my first chapter in my first chapter book
- I got my very first publishing contract
- I helped save a person's life today on the operating table
- I helped a family keep their home from foreclosure
- My baby took his or her first steps
- I successfully completed my first science experiment
- I began to read today for the first time
- I got my first A on a Math test ever
- I may not have scored the highest on my SATs but I did much better than last time
- I made another rent or mortgage or credit card payment
- I changed my first tire today
- I made time to spend with my kids today or this week(end)
- I remembered my wife's and my anniversary and said "happy anniversary, honey" first
- My spouse and I are making progress in couple's counseling
- I wrote the first draft of my first screenplay
- I am preparing to take my first step toward conquering my fear
- I did a good job ministering to that couple today
- My team and I saved a house from burning to the ground
- I completed my first scene as an actor and got really good feedback from my coach
- I was able to talk to my patient and help them through some difficult medical news
- I went for a walk today
- My friend and I did a good job painting the house this weekend
- I followed a pattern or a recipe and I am creating my first piece of clothing or baked item
- I paid my taxes in full this month
- We have started a savings fund for our retirement
- We have opened a bank account for our children

- I took time for me this afternoon
- I did a good deed for someone else
- I am volunteering for a charitable organization
- My spouse and I worked on our marriage today
- I wrote a letter to a person I was angry with and then threw it away

You see, when we celebrate the little wins, we feel better, we work better and we look forward to more opportunities where we can reward ourselves and others. This increase in serotonin (the happy chemical) in our brain causes such a wonderful little surge and we can keep that going because it is good and healthy to allow ourselves to do this. There are already so many things out there vying to bring us down, why not take the time to create this little but significant space of happiness for ourselves?

So now, think about it and jot down some little wins you have experienced on your road to success. Jot them down here or do so in your own journal. Remember, this is something you will want to come back to and refer to again and again because these will help be reminders and motivation for future successes through future challenging times:

Remembering to Congratulate Others

Whether it's your child who got a spot on the school athletics team or your spouse who completed their budget and got it approved at work, or a neighbor who won a prize for his or her garden, it is vital to remember to congratulate others on their wins. This reminds them that you care, that you are paying attention, that you want the best for them and that you are their cheerleader in their corner just as much as you may like them to be a cheerleader in your corner. It is so important to make sure that we take the time to do this in our day, so if it means putting in the reminder on your phone calendar that today is the day of your kid's game or the day your spouse has that big meeting, a little gesture and remembering a person and what they are dealing with in their day goes a long way.

One spouse said to me "*It means the world to me when my husband celebrates my little wins, whether it's baking a delicious set of brownies for our kid's school bake sale or doing a great job in my work presentation, it means the world to me when he just sends me a text and encourages me. It really helps to strengthen our relationship and helps to make our bond that much tighter, and even our kids subconsciously pick up on that when they are watching mommy and daddy. It makes me appreciate him that much more.*"

One child said "*I wish my mom would make time for me in her day. She is so busy with her job and with making money that she totally forgets me and all the things I'm going through in my day. I need her support.*" This child did have a conversation with her parent upon a professional's suggestion and after just two meetings, she shared this with me: "*My mom is almost a totally different person. Now, she turns off her phone at 9 pm and makes sure that she spends the rest of the night focused on just me. When we talked about things in counseling, I told her how her being so busy made me feel bad and unimportant and I'm thankful that she heard me and decided to change her ways. We now talk all the time and she makes way more time for* me, which I need and appreciate. It also makes me want to make time for her too."

Another spouse said "*He used to not pay attention to me and then I made it a point to set aside time each day to connect. We do this in front of the television but nonetheless, we do it. I explained to him how I want to be heard and how we aren't connecting and thankfully, he heard me and decided to do something about it. We now make sure that each evening, we spend time connecting and we spend time listening to each other. It's more than just 'family time', it's a necessary time to connect and to make our bond stronger. We now celebrate these little wins by going out once a month for gelato.*"

As you can see from these people, this is time well spent and in the end, makes both of you or all of you stronger, better people. It is also important to invite Christ into your family and sharing time, allowing Him to speak to you each individually as you enjoy.

20

Speak It!

This is such an important topic, I felt it deserved its own chapter.

The power of the spoken word. In Scripture (Proverbs 18:21), it says that **"life and death are in the power of the tongue."** This means that we can cause good things to happen with the words we speak, just like we can cause bad things to happen with the words we speak. Either way, we are causing something to happen so why not cause good (or, the best) things to happen? We have to recognize and accept this fact and as such, be very mindful of the words we choose to speak. Yes, we can get frustrated and use curse words or speak negatively, such as *"Oh man, this situation is never going to get better"* but that's when you need to stop yourself and you need to change your words.

> **As creatures of habit, we have to remind ourselves to speak positively continually.**

Because humans are creatures of habit, we have to make sure that we are training ourselves to speak positively consistently. I often find that when people start to do this (myself included) we can dedicate ourselves to doing it for a day or two or ten but then when we don't see the immediate results, we stop doing it and we go back to our old habits, starting to speak negatively again. We need to stop that and we need to train ourselves to do better, consistently. Put reminders for yourself on your phone, write reminders for yourself in your home, put the reminders in your car or on your streaming devices, write it everywhere and anywhere you would like. Just do it and eventually, it will become a part of your routine.

This does apply for when things are getting challenging as well. We have to stay dedicated to speaking positively and to inviting good into our lives.

Here are some examples of how we can speak positively over our lives:

* I am working hard and succeeding at work
* We are doing a great job on this case and we are making great headway
* I am dedicating myself to my relationship and spending time cherishing my spouse
* I am treating others with love and care and I am receiving the same in return
* Good breaks find me
* My family and friends make me a priority and I make them a priority too
* I am getting into the schools of my choice
* Timing and luck favor me and work in my favor
* I am being recognized for being a great

----

* I am positive and work hard in all I do
* My children are on the right course and will stay on the right course
* My marriage is thriving each and every day
* My spouse and I make time for each other and we connect

* My weight loss and fitness goals are going very well and I am making great headway
* I am on track to make partner at my law firm
* The medical report may not be great but God has the last and final word
* We are saving for our first house and blessings will find us to find the right one
* I am finding favor with the Lord
* I am taking a wonderful vacation with my family
* The Lord is helping us pay our bills easily and effortlessly
* All the right doors are opening for me / us
* My family and I are taking steps to remain close
* I am meeting the love of my life and we are getting married
* I don't see a way but the Lord has ways I don't know about yet
* God loves me and cherishes me, even when others don't
* I am getting the promotion at work
* Money and wealth and abundance come to me easily and effortlessly
* We are going to have the happiest Christmas or Easter or Lent
* The Lord is helping me stay strong during my fast so I can complete it successfully
* I am donating to this charitable organization and pray that the Lord multiplies the good that this money does in the lives of those it touches
* The Lord helps me pay my tithes
* I am beautiful, smart and one of a kind
* I am handsome, smart and amazing
* People respect me and appreciate me everywhere I go
* We are able to afford and go on lovely vacations
* I look and feel great, at any age
* My body and my mind are healthy, happy and alert at all ages
* My spouse and I are in the best place ever

One of the most important things to remember is that even when you say these words, challenges will still come. Does that mean we should stop? Certainly not. If we stop speaking empowering words every time we encounter opposition, we will not get very far. Whenever we encounter opposition, we can ask the Lord to help us through the opposition and to make things easier. We also need to continue working hard and speaking the most empowering words with faith and conviction.

Speaking empowering, life-affirming words works for literally every area of our lives.

A lady I know was nearing her senior years and began speaking negatively over her life. "*I am old. I am past my prime. It's over for me.*" I can't tell you how many times I asked her to be more mindful of her words, to speak positively over her life and to speak life-affirming words over herself and her spouse. I provided examples, I provided literature on this but unfortunately, she refused to do so. Now, about five years since this negativity began, she looks much older, has many more wrinkles, is generally a much more negative person and she generally feels tired and out of breath most of the time. Unfortunately, this is a trend that once the negative words begin, it takes time to reverse the process. More on this in the next section.

Get The Ball Rolling

In reality, it takes a good amount of time for the ball to get rolling in the right direction; for positive things to begin happening after we speak the life-affirming words. It also takes time for things to manifest here on earth so even if you say "*I am receiving large amounts of good health and good fortune*", you will not likely see them drop into your lap instantly. It takes time to get the ball rolling and for good things to start replacing negative things but the best thing you can do is to get it rolling and to start moving things into the right direction. You see, I say "replacing the negative" because when we don't start speaking positive words, negativity comes into play. We don't have to invite negativity - it will find us. This is a broken world and as such, that negativity does come and so it's almost like we have to fight it so that it doesn't take hold or take root.

So, get the ball rolling in the right direction by speaking positively and speaking words of faith. Most people know quite well that life can be difficult (and sometimes, very difficult) but what you don't want is to surround yourself with people who will influence you to start or to continue that negativity. I have had to lessen time with some people in my life who were unfortunately being quite negative, and they would not stop. **People who are successful in life are not those to whom nothing bad happens. They are people who are able to see past the negative circumstances and are able to see the positive despite the negative circumstances.** It is refreshing to watch videos or to hear testimonials of successful, positive people who have overcome great odds to get to where they are today. People who are in all different fields and who came from families in poverty, who have experienced tremendous and debilitating illnesses, language barriers, bankruptcy, had every door slam in their face, and more, yet, they broke through in faith and they are now reaping the rewards of their action, steadfastness and of their faith.

One Christian author I find particularly inspiring is Nick Vujicic, the man who has no legs or arms and who works each day as a Motivational Speaker and Evangelist. This man does not have the everyday use of his arms or legs and yet, he is able to preach motivation, the goodness of God and is able to convey to people the hope that they long for. He looks past his own challenges and sees the positive and aims to evoke that in others too. Somebody else could easily have taken that and could have been terribly negative, wishing only negative on others because they feel that they have been very hard done by and that life has been incredibly unfair to them.

When we realize how good God has already been to us (no matter your circumstances), God has given each of us so much and loves us. It is then up to us to come to Him in thanksgiving and to seek what good things He has in store for us because no matter who you are, where you are from, what color your skin is, how much money is in your bank account, or anything else, He has great things in store for you.

One of the Greatest Tests

One of my favorite pastors, Joyce Meyer, said in one of her videos that one of the greatest tests is how we treat others when we are going through difficulties. I think this is very well said. When things are difficult in our lives, especially for a sustained amount of time, and we are getting rocked by things, and we feel we are being stretched, it can be very hard to treat people well or kindly. It can be hard to not have people get on your nerves, especially when we have many other things on our minds. When we are going through such times, we have to take time to love ourselves, to be good to ourselves in whatever ways we would like and are realistic, and that does not have to mean very expensive or very cumbersome things. The littlest happiness can mean so much and can go a very long way to causing ourselves to feel better. It's all about the attitude with which we approach things and we must also remember that we can and should pray for the Lord to give us strength for the things we are going through.

I am including here a suggested prayer that you may feel you want to pray, either in your mind or out loud. The purpose of this prayer is to provide anyone with the words to use when we want to pray to the Lord for His strength and His goodness. One of the reasons I am including suggested prayers in this book is because I think it can be very helpful for people (no matter where you are in your walk with God) to read the prayers that other people have prayed and that can be helpful to us in our walk and in drawing on the Lord's goodness and strength. Here is the prayer for strength. Of course, you are more than welcome to tweak it as you need to, as per your situation and context.

"Lord Jesus, I love You. You know that I am, right now, going through some difficulties (feel free to name those difficulties). Not only do I ask You to give me Your wisdom in this (what I need to learn here) but I also pray for You to deliver me from this in Your way and in Your time. I pray for Your strength as I go through these things and for Your to show me the ways through. You do not bring anything to Your children unless You have a very good purpose for it, so I am praying that You reveal those purposes to me and let me pass through these times. In Jesus' name. Amen."

21

Tech and Other Good Things

I love tech. The eases, conveniences and advantages that it provides us are wonderful, beneficial and life-altering. But like with any other thing, we have to know how to use it properly.

I started off not knowing or understanding technology but quickly realized that I would need to learn it and understand for school and for life, and then once I got the basic grasp of it for those reasons, I started to really enjoy using it and loving the benefits it can provide. We can send something in a fraction of a moment to someone on the other side of the world, we can communicate seamlessly and in real time with anyone, anywhere and at any time. We can send payments to anyone for any reason, we can create documents and spreadsheets at ease and depending on the program you use, without even hitting a "save" button, you can create lengthy and amazing documents, and much more.

Tech is changing all of our lives in every way and one of my favorite questions is when people ask me if God ever intended us to have and to use technology. The answer is of course He wanted us to use it, but in the right ways. God is always for the advancement of people and for allowing for things that will help us and benefit us. Technology has afforded people so many conveniences, luxuries, etc., including social media uses to connect people and to bring people together, to share, to engage community, and much more and we are wisest when we use it well and for the right purposes. I still find it awesome that people use it to Facetime call each other, to connect and communicate by email, to send things halfway across the world, and more.

Some fantastic uses of technology include:

- Call and message loved ones
- Send pictures to one another
- Send complicated but important documents
- Send jokes and funnies
- Watch or stream television and movies
- Find better ways to do something (ex. vacuum technology)
- Use messaging to let loved ones know you care about them
- Cars and motor vehicles
- Using the radio for news, entertainment, education and much more
- Providing people with access to resources when they otherwise would not have had that access
- Better construction & design of everything from buildings and transportation and far beyond
- More and better access to educational programs and schools

When it comes to how tech can be used to bring you God's best, He will use the advent of technologies to achieve and accomplish His purposes in your life and in the lives of others. God always likes to bring you and others the maximum benefit of anything He gives you and so from online purchasing and ease of connecting to community and dissemination of Pastoral sermons, there are many good uses for the collective term of tech.

For instance, we can be in Canada (where this book was written) and we can enjoy a sermon recorded elsewhere in the world and live streamed or via uploaded video. We can complete a document and we can email it to anyone, anywhere in the world and within seconds, they will get it. We can find the community and the support we are looking for and can connect with other community members anywhere in the world and talk about things that we are experiencing, and find support in other people going through the same things. One of the best things about the widespread use of tech is the fact that it directly caters to something we know that is in our heart and for which we are built: community and fellowship.

* Take the example of the family that just lost a loved one and see how a community can both help them heal and help them connect with others who have been through similar things.
* Take the young child who is looking for friends in the midst of a pandemic and desperately wants to talk to others who may be going through the same thing.
* Take the elderly person who wants to see their children or grandchildren or great-grandchildren halfway across the world and can use technology to do that.
* Take people who are looking for a beautiful vacation and so they hop onto a flight and go somewhere warm in the middle of a snowstorm where they live.
* Take a business deal that will provide a person or a family much-needed money for themselves and great seeds for their tithes and that requires signatures that need to happen quickly and effectively.
* Take the dissemination and organization of lifesaving MRI machines, x-ray machines and other medical devices that are invaluable in the world.
* Take the use of planes to get much-needed food and medicine to remote countries where help and medical attention are needed.
* Consider the uses of power that are used to heat and to provide electricity that warm a home and help a family stay warm and healthy during those blisteringly cold winter months.

Tech has so many important, life-saving uses and needs to be used in the right ways. We would be very wise to pray for how else we can use technology to further new advances, new inventions, and new ways of making life for humanity better.

Helping The Environment

Technology also has tools to help and heal the environment. I strongly believe that our world would be in much worse condition than we already are in if we didn't have technology to help create new and better ways of managing garbage, recycling, re-packaging, and using human waste to create new advances that would actually help humanity.

Another amazing thing about tech is how quickly and rapidly it allows us to move, change, and adapt. There have been wonderful inventions that have been and continue to be invaluable to the environment and that are completely tech-based and use resources in nature that we already have readily available. Without technology, the pushing of envelopes on what tech can do and the amazing visions of the people who followed their vision and did something about creating these pieces, we (and by we I mean mankind) would not be the beneficiary of the wonderful things that we have at our disposal today. God always gives visions to people to help us do wonderful things, things that will be grand in making the world a better place but it's up to the people who are receiving the vision to take strategic, God-directed actions on those visions for mankind to see its best from it.

Of course God wants the best for us....He has been showing us that since the Garden.

Negative Uses

Technology does also have its negative uses. We can misuse technology to allow, facilitate or encourage such negative things as porn, gambling, facilitating of extra-marital affairs, the dissemination of murder, violence and forcible sex, human trafficking and much more. This wonderful tool in the wrong hands can be a real recipe for disaster, as we have already seen far too often in the world. People need to be and to remain alert to these terrible things, otherwise we could unintentionally fall into any one of them and get ourselves on the road to some very dangerous, deceptive and addictive practices.

An older gentleman I know confided that he was dealing with some pornographic issues. He had said that he tried to turn it off but it was proving to be more and more difficult than he had thought it would be. He had said that it was becoming a problem because he was finding himself hiding it from his wife, whom he loved, and didn't want it to hurt her or their marriage but he was finding that each time he was alone at home, he would turn to that for his viewing needs. Fast forward several months and this man had to really pray his way through and lean on the strength and wisdom provided by the Holy Spirit in order to beat what was becoming an addiction. As he continued to pray, he slowly started seeing himself waning off of the videos, allowing himself to replace the images of the women in the videos with images and thoughts of his wife instead. He shared with me that in this time of recovery, that many significant challenges were presenting themselves and he found that, in the end, he needed to talk to his wife about this and to get her support too. I encouraged him to do so because this is what he felt he needed in order to move past this; he opened up to his wife about this and they began to work through it together.

Controlling Ourselves

I say this with all due respect: As humans with free will, we can sometimes allow ourselves to get stuck in very destructive practices. These practices then eventually become habits and then because these snuck up on you, you may not even realize it until much later that it is a full-blown habit, routine or addiction. As such, we need to pray for God's wisdom in knowing the look-for's and to how we can protect ourselves from things like online gambling, excessive video gaming, pills, alcohol, porn and more that may seem innocent on the surface but are anything but.

When left unchecked and untreated, these things have not only the potential but the likelihood of destroying individual lives, families, and on a much larger scale, contributing to the breakdown of society. For example, when you have one family man that is dealing with, say, alcohol addiction and becomes a mean drunk when he returns home, the impact on his family life will undoubtedly be bad. His children will see this, they will be exposed to one of daddy's episodes, and you can imagine the havoc it would wreak on his life, work and marriage. He may stop going to Church, stop praying, stop talking to or opening up to his spouse, start shunning his kids and open the door for terrible consequences. On a larger scale, if this happens to 10% or 12% of the men in our population, we will have so many destroyed relationships, shattered families, uptick in divorces, downtick in Church attendance, children who have grown up watching daddy drink and possibly verbally or physically abuse them, etc. This is a recipe for the slow but sure breakdown of society.

When we take our eyes off of Jesus, we will eventually be led down the wrong path and we will have to eventually redirect ourselves to Jesus and to the values our society holds dear. The more people stay away from God, the more we deviate from the teachings of Scripture, the more we deny the teachings of Scripture and the solid values it outlines, and the more we take on the stance that "we know better", the more we are going to be led to our downfall, and to society's downfall. Following Jesus and doing what He says through the promptings of the Holy Spirit is not always easy. Please trust me when I say that I have wanted to do many things that the Holy Spirit guided me away from and it did not feel good at first. In fact it was downright painful. **I understand**

now how following His promptings was the right thing to do and how it ultimately benefited me.

To give you a for instance, after my ex and I broke up many years ago, I contemplated getting back together with him and had the opportunity to do so. The Holy Spirit was telling me a very different thing, though, which did not feel good to my flesh. I did obey and it was only weeks later that I found that, in fact, during our entire relationship, he had been cheating on me with different women and that he had consistently lied to me. It makes sense, therefore, that getting back together with him would not have been a great idea because of my value system that I deserve a man who will remain faithful to me. Does this mean that if you don't already have a relationship with Christ, that you deserve for bad relationships and bad things to happen to you? Certainly not. We all deserve to have great treatment in any relationship just as much as we deserve to provide the great treatment, but my point is that being a daughter of God provides an added reminder that Jesus died to give you a good, healthy, happy life.

Going back to my point about technology: it is when I read many Facebook posts about God's will from Christian community groups that allowed the Holy Spirit to speak to me and advised me that this was not the right person for me. Did the posts tell me that directly? Of course not. Instead, the post read "Grace is how you let go of something that was never intended for you" and I knew right then (through the promptings of the Holy Spirit) that this quote was speaking directly to my former relationship and that this man was not the right one for me.

Romantic Relationships & Being Online

Many times in our day and age, women and men will both go online in search of love. There are Christian websites that say that they will help you find God's mate for you but when you look further into the site, many of the company's practices directly negate God's values as stated in Scripture.

Going online can be an absolutely wonderful way to meet and to come together with your spouse but each situation is unique and I encourage you to pray and to ask Him *"Is this where the man or woman You have intended to be my husband or my wife will be found?"* He will reply. He will guide you. And it will save you a lot of time, frustration, energy, effort and money. If he or she isn't online (or at least not on the website you are considering registering on) then you will meet many people and ultimately, it will be an exercise in frustration because the bottom line is: the right person isn't there and you could have better spent that time elsewhere, looking in the right places.

I won't forget how years ago (before I had started my walk with the Lord), I considered hiring a matchmaker upon the advice of a friend who did not have any walk with God. She suggested I hire this matchmaker and "get things on the road". I decided to check it out and gave this matchmaker a call. She explained high and low what she would do for me, the personality assessments, this, that and the other. She also informed me that she charged a hefty $15,000 for the service. I promptly excused myself from the conversation and hung up. Looking back, I am very grateful that I didn't use these services because this lady had no walk with God and was obviously not going to lead me correctly. She would lead me to someone (maybe even many) but the process would have been futile - he wouldn't have been the one God intended. God does that exact same service of matchmaking (and much more) and He doesn't even charge you a penny. He will also be there through all your dates, helping you understand your love and He will be there with you both throughout your marriage, helping you both each step of the way.

Christian Prayer & Teaching Apps

There are a number of wonderful apps that you can download if you have a smartphone and an internet connection that will provide free, regular access to sermons that provide wonderful and well-explained interpretations of the Bible. The apps that are out there are by some of the most renowned Pastors and Preachers, and cover every different possible area of life from careers to relationships and much more. All of the apps have a myriad of ways with which you can connect with them and ways to download their messages, stream them, and they are generally made available free of charge. Here are some of my absolute favorites:

- John Hagee
- Chip Ingram
- Joyce Meyer
- Charles Stanley
- Joel Osteen
- Jurgen Matthesius
- Billy Graham
- Andy Stanley
- Charles Windoll
- John MacArthur

With the beauty of technology and the amazing levels of accessibility we all enjoy today, downloading and listening with an open heart and an open mind is easier today than it has ever been.

Remember that when you are listening to the sermons, to ask the Holy Spirit to really talk to you, helping you to understand what is being explained in a deeper, more meaningful way and a way that will help the information really settle on your mind and in your heart.

Volunteering and Giving of your Time

One of the best gifts we can ever give is your time. Volunteering at

Church, a bookstore, or a charitable organization is not only deeply satisfying but it would be much appreciated by the organization to whom you are providing the help. It is really amazing how anyone these days can, without even leaving the comfort of their home, can easily give of their time, their talents, their skills and their expertise using online resources. Reach out to any of the organizations you would like to and offer your help either online or face to face.

Tech is a great tool, dear reader, but it has to be used in the right ways and has to further your own personal relationship with the Lord.

22

Your Ministry

I am going to spend a bit of time here talking about your Ministry. Ministry means that thing that God has put on your heart to do for the purposes of the greater good of society. For some, it could be an entrepreneurship Ministry, for others, a teaching Ministry, for others, a praying Ministry and platform, etc. We are all called to some sort of Ministry, or we may be called to help and support a Ministry.

Your Ministry, regardless of what it is, has tremendous importance to God, to people, to the world. Your Ministry will correspond to and will be based on your talent and your skills because God always equips us with all we need to do His good works and for the benefit of His Kingdom. We have to remember that what we do here on earth is tremendously important in the Heavenly realm and has to be in compliance with what He calls us to do. **A Ministry is a calling and He will give you the tools you will need to fulfill that calling.**

Ask Him & Structure

When you are working on your Ministry, you must: a) seek Him and His help b) ask Him if you are on the right track c) pray that you are using the resources in the right ways   d) check-in with Him to have everything line up perfectly.

Now, one of the things I learned the hard way is that Ministries do evolve and do change. In other words, they will likely change and evolve as they grow over time. It is really important that when you are setting up your Ministry, that you do so in the right way, regardless of where you are around the world. For instance, one of my old professors mentioned that she had to set things up and structured her Ministry under certain categories, given that any other category meant that the government would have control over what she covers in her teaching Ministry and would have the authorization to shut her down should she deviate from that mandate. This is something she wanted to clearly and definitely avoid because another person's agenda and mandate for her Ministry could be totally different from what God has called her to do and that would defeat the entire purpose of her having started her Ministry.

Challenges & Seeking Him

We also have to remember that as with anything else, we are going to experience challenges and when those challenges arise, we have to seek Him. The challenges that come will not be a surprise to Him in any way, so we have to seek Him and ask Him about the things that will be coming up. It is so important to make sure that we are following each thing that He guides us to and that we have......COURAGE.....

Courage

What do I mean by courage and why do I have a separate section for it? Starting your own Ministry takes courage. You are looking at a commitment of time, money, energy and effort that will need to be dedicated to this and it is a considerable entrepreneurial endeavor. All of that requires courage. In addition, having the courage to put your God-given skill set out there - to invite people to partake, to learn from, to feast on the gifts that God has given you, to benefit and to grow from it in ways that as this point, you may only just be able to imagine - all of that takes courage too. It is vitally important to have "khutzpah" to do the things God has called us to do.

I will give you a "for instance": A lady I knew who was tremendously gifted in Christ and whose closeness to Christ was exemplary, in my opinion, knew that she was being called to a teaching and prayer Ministry. I encouraged her to get started, to work on her website, to do the things she knew God had put on her heart to do and to enjoy the process. I offered my services to help her in any way that I could and I offered her some strategies that I could tell would work for her based on her innate "tough and wise girl" skill set. She was a natural for so many of the things that she was called to do and I would talk to her about them often. As time went on, the prayer meetings didn't get scheduled, the site didn't get built and certainly, she wasn't using the time and the initiative that God was putting at her disposal to do what was needed. I asked her what was going on and she simply said (and I paraphrase) "Who am I to do this? I can't do these things." I tried to explain how good she was at leading people to Christ and how much she had to offer but she would not relent. Today, the website is not built, and nothing has been done. She is leading a happy life today as a wife and mother and that's fantastic but she did not do as the Lord guided back then and that is unfortunate for all the people who would have benefited tremendously from all the good that would have been borne out of her Ministry.

> Readers, it does take courage. It does take resources. It does take persistence but God put that greatness inside of you. Everything you need to do what He has called you to do is already in you. I hope you will answer the call when it comes.

Allow me to offer you this prayer:

"I pray for the Lord to speak clearly into your heart, to show you in words and in images/visuals what He wants for you, and how and when you are to do it. Let Him speak directly into your heart so that you understand His love for you, His love for the Ministry He is calling you to take on, how and when He wants you to take this on and let Him lead you down the path to being able to do this for the Kingdom. May He make you steadfast in your faith and may He shine your feet with His light so that your steps are clear and succinct, and may He cause others to pray for you and for your Ministry as you walk with Him, as you undertake strategic decisions, as you put in your resources into this and certainly, as challenges arise. May your Ministry be just as He wants it and may it positively touch and affect people around the world. In Jesus' name. Amen."

23

The Inconvenient Moments

In any Ministry (in any endeavor, really) you will have inconvenient moments. You will have moments where you are called to do things that are inconvenient or inconveniently-timed. You could be interrupted during dinner to take a business phone call, a work email can come through at a time that is inconvenient, you received a wonderful speaking opportunity but it falls on your child's birthday, you are asked to put in money for promotions and advertising but you already feel stretched paying your family's bills. We all experience those difficult, inconvenient moments and I empathize, they can be so hard.

I remember in the time I was writing this book, I had to miss many dinners with my family and lots of time I could have been doing something else but because the thoughts were running, things were rolling, and there was much to be done for a good book to be produced, I needed to dedicate myself to this book and to my other books, among the many other things that need to be done in life. I had to put in money to publish my books and I was already considerably financially extended, but I chose to spend hours and hours at my laptop. They are sacrifices. In order to do great things, we do have to sacrifice. We do have to make time for our endeavors and to ask God to open up the doors to allow us to have the time, money and resources to do the things that need to be done.

I sometimes look at Olympians, such as Michael Phelps and Sunisa Lee - of course there are many, many more but those two are two that come to mind right now - and I see how much passion, dedication, focus and drive they have to accomplish leadership status within an Olympic circle. That in my opinion, is the creme de la creme. They have sacrificed countless hours in the pool and in the gym, respectively, working on their craft, honing their expertise, eating right, sleeping right, not going out to party with friends, and the many, many, many hours of practice they obviously endured. **When I need a reality check and begin to complain about how much time and effort I put into something or I need to put into something, I think about Olympians like them and I am amazed. I enjoy looking at the example of those who have done such tremendous things, amazing accomplishments and while I am in awe, I also use it to propel me to put my best into what I am doing.**

When God calls you to do something, He knows it's going to be inconvenient at times but He's asking you to do it anyway. He's asking you to trust Him and to put your best into what you are doing. He's asking you to let Him guide you. I can tell you unequivocally and without reservation that He guided me through every single step of writing this book, from when I should write, to the thoughts and main points I should include, to the chapter and section headings and subheadings, all of it. He guided me to do each step. I certainly had those days or those times when I didn't feel like doing it. I just wanted to sit in front of the television and veg out, or I wanted to go out and have fun, but I knew that doing that would mean that I don't get a great chapter written, I don't get that thought put to "paper", I don't help someone on their walk with Christ and I wouldn't be putting my own very best into being the kind of author I want to be and that I know God has called me to be, and that people would not benefit from reading about these things and my experiences.

I'd like to take this moment to ask you to pause and reflect on the sacrifices you have made in your life previously that have led you to the successes and accomplishments you have and enjoy today. What did you give up? Take your time and think about this because it will be used to fuel your future endeavors, to give you the sometimes much-needed motivation to pursue the things you feel God has put on your heart today. Remember to use your journal when needed so you can have a record of this and look back on it again and again. You can use the space provided to answer this question or write about it in your journal, phone or somewhere else.

Sharing Can Be Hard

Sharing can be really inconvenient. Sharing means that we are opening ourselves up to others, allowing them to read and to know about our lives and yes, we open ourselves up to their possible criticism and judgments.

When we all share and put out thoughts, ideas, testimonials and opinions "out there", we are sharing and we are opening ourselves up to judgments and criticism. Some people might think that what we are doing is great and they may give us praise (which is always wonderful) and some may try to tear us down with mean-spirited, nasty and judgmental comments. Any way you slice it, just like that young kid who gets up in class and reads his or her book report or his or her short story to the class and faces the looks, judgments and possibly criticism of the class, we are opening ourselves up to those criticisms and that can be very hard.

So what do we do about that? Do we stop sharing altogether?

We can share with the world or with a few that we choose to but we have to make sure we are sharing wisely. God shows us how much to share, when to share, with whom to share, why we share that and how to respond to criticism when it comes.

For instance, God will never ask you to air out your proverbial "dirty laundry" in front of others, to embarrass or humiliate yourself. He will never ask you to do things that are humiliating. He loves you too much to do that and He will never ask you to sensationalize your "dirty laundry".

Remember also that you are strong in Christ so any criticism that comes can just roll off your back and does not have to affect you. "**My peace I give to you**" (John 14:27) is what Jesus offers in the Bible, and it's no less true today than it was back then.

The Dinnertime Phone Call

I remember listening to a very famous film producer speak at a conference. He and his entire family were there because his business had turned into a family business and so his wife and children were also there and were clearly on the producing journey and path with him. They talked about how they would be trying to get everything together, funding together for a movie and that they would be just about to sit down to dinner and a phone call would come saying that someone had stepped out of the project and they were now $15 million short of the budget needed for the film and how they would need to deal with that and talk it over together, seeing now what they could do to make up that difference because otherwise their project won't get made. It was inconvenient, troublesome (having $15 million taken out of your project is no laughing matter) and I bet that made their dinnertime conversation topic take a mighty turn.

That Tuition

When we speak about the inconvenient moments, one of the most universally expensive items to purchase is tuition. This is something that families (certainly parents or guardians) stress over and try their best to prepare for over the years and because they know this mammoth expense is coming for their kid's or ward's education. Whether it's private school education, university or college tuition, you know it's going to cost a lot. This inconvenience requires forward-planning, sacrifice, hard work, strategic planning and control (I say control because you could go and spend your kid's tuition money on random things but you will need to control yourself).

Success is going to present those inconvenient moments and we will have to deal with them when they come up but we also know that we can rely on the goodness of God to help us through and to help resolve the issue.

A lady I met had wanted to start a Ministry and she was very excited about it. She felt very sure that God put the idea for this Ministry on her heart and while she didn't have the money for its startup, she knew that if it was His will, that the money would come. So she began praying for it. Slowly, the money began trickling in from different places and in different amounts but it did and when I talked to her about it, she was just so pleased but what I found interesting is that she was not at all surprised. She was very happy about it but not at all surprised because she told me that she knew it was God's will for her to do this and therefore, the money would start coming in. I find it simply amazing and wonderfully refreshing when people of strong faith don't worry, don't fret and don't stress but are so sure that this is what God has brought them that they continue the tasks they know they need to do, fully remaining in faith that the resource will appear and then sure enough, it does. How rewarding!

Weathering It When the Timing Is Tight

Something that can make things a little nerve-wracking sometimes is God's timing. God is never late but He is also not early. He is on time. This means that He isn't usually early in the sense that we would like our problems taken care of today, and not "in time". So how do we weather this? How do we handle it when the timing is a bit tight in our opinion or viewpoint and we are sitting there, waiting intently for our blessing to come through?

Well, you could do the following:

Pray for His comfort
Pray for His wisdom and
Rely on His character

I will explain each. 1. Praying for Him to comfort you during a difficult time is wise and Biblical - we are asking Him to supernaturally let us know that He has this problem in the palm of His hand and that He is capable. 2. Praying for His wisdom will give us God's perspective on the problem and He will show how He is not late, but He is on time. You may think the due date for something must be on such-and-such date, but that isn't necessarily the case. 3. Relying on His character means that you know He is going to come through because He does not just "drop" His children or any that come to Him.

Let me provide some examples of what I mean here:

A mother had an athlete son and they were waiting for his scholarship offer to come in, in order to pay for university. Her son had been an athlete for years and they were relying on the tuition money for him. Time was passing and the scholarship offers were not forthcoming. She was beginning to get a little nervous and she kept in her mind that the tuition payment would be due on a particular day. She knew that God had spoken into her spirit that the money would be there but because the deadline for tuition payment was nearing quickly, and they had not received the money, she and the family were getting nervous. They considered taking a loan but knew that that would need to be repaid and with interest so they didn't feel that was a good option for them because they didn't have the funds to do that. She knew in her spirit the money would come but she admitted that the waiting period was hard and she mentioned that she wishes that she had prayed for more comfort and peace of mind at that time. The day the tuition money was due, they received an offer for a scholarship that was ten times the amount of the tuition money. The scholarship would cover tuition, books, housing, ancillary expenses and much more. It was the offer they had been waiting for and it came on the same day the tuition was due. Did God come through? Yes, He did.

A girl I know I will call Catie knew that God had put it on her heart that she was not to go back to her old job. She had outgrown the position and the company and this was no longer where God intended her to be but no other employment offers were forthcoming. She was totally puzzled and didn't understand. She had worked her whole adult life so she was confused about what she was supposed to do, where the money was going to come from. She decided to remain in faith about it. She knew that God was going to come through and was going to do something amazing in her life. She was aware that God knew where her finances were and the payments she had to make. So, without seeing the whole proverbial staircase, she decided to stay in faith and see how God provides. When she talked about this before the miracle happened, she was a little nervous and that nervousness came through in her voice. Sure enough, a phone call came that had the potential to change her circumstances. Because she was so nervous, she prayed a silent prayer saying that she would be staying quiet during the phone call and that she would let the Lord take over and bring her His blessing. Sure enough, after she said what she needed to say when the person was asking her, she stayed totally quiet and at the end of the call, she discovered that she would be receiving significantly more in her pay than she thought she would be. For weeks after that call, she would remember that call and how much God had provided and that sure enough, what she had heard in her spirit was true. God had provided and she was very grateful.

Yet another example of an inconvenience (and this is a case of life and death so read with a little bit of caution in knowing that ahead of time) and of God providing was in the case of Gerry. Gerry had had undiagnosed heart problems in his life. He had a few different health issues and these were obviously making life more difficult. One afternoon, his family found him passed out and unconscious, on the ground outside and not breathing or moving. Understandably, his family began panicking and trying to revive him. A doctor who happened to be in the area noticed and was trying to resuscitate him and was pounding on his chest in the right ways to revive him but nothing was working. In the corner where nobody could see her, his niece prayed a silent prayer asking the Lord to forgive Gerry's sins and if it is his time to go, let him go in peace but making it also clear that his family did not want to lose him. The doctor pounded on his chest relentlessly, doing his best to revive Gerry but nothing was working. Finally the ambulance came and took Gerry to the hospital on a stretcher. A few hours later, they had gotten word that Gerry was ok, he had been revived and doctors said that the chances of Gerry having come out of that cardiac episode without severe brain damage was less than 2%. Gerry was exceptionally lucky and his niece told him afterward about how she had prayed for him and how God had saved him.

Readers, these are all inconvenient moments, yes, but it is in the inconvenience that God can show up big time. It is in those inconvenient moments that we can see God's goodness and provision and while inconvenient, it makes us rely on Him more and that is something He wants us to do. In the Bible, God has always indicated that He wants us to rely on Him and to draw from His provision. I go back to the fact that we are sheep and we need His Shepherding to get us through.

Jana had moved to Canada in hopes of a better future for herself and her family. When she arrived, she was obviously scared, felt a little bit lost, and was unsure of how she would make it. She had no other family other than the ones who came with her so there was no apartment, work, infrastructure set up for her to benefit from when she got here. She did, however, stumble luckily on the Peoples Church at Bayview and Sheppard in Toronto. Through this Christ-centered Church, she found a very welcoming community, she found some very helpful resources and she found a job. She was so very grateful to have found this resource at a time in her life when she and her family desperately needed the help, the warmth, the love and the comfort of Christ and of community. You may also be surprised to discover that when Jana and her family moved here, they were not Christian. They had heard talk of Jesus but had never turned to Him, and knew very little about Him. You see, the Peoples' Church has a beautiful outreach program for non-Christians where they can come, they can enjoy community and fellowship and they can learn about the help and the love that is available in Christ. Jana and her family could see how loving this community was and on their own, they made the decision to accept Christ as their Savior and Provider. Jana and her family now go to Peoples each week for fellowship, praise and worship and love that they have found Christ.

Are all of these examples of success and abundance? You absolutely better believe it.

My last example in this chapter of inconvenient moments is that of Norma. Norma was not a believer and she had found herself pregnant and alone. Her family had turned their backs and the father of the baby didn't want anything to do with her anymore. Norma was devastated, alone and pregnant with a real lack of resources. She needed help and she wanted to be sure that she was doing the right thing for herself and for her baby. She had heard of the Pregnancy Care Center in Toronto and decided to check it out. She didn't want to terminate the pregnancy but she didn't have the resources to sustain this on her own so she was looking for help and for love and a lot of both. She visited the Pregnancy Care Center where she learned about the love and care of the Lord. Norma was very reluctant at first because she hadn't grown up knowing Jesus and frankly, to her at that point, she saw Him as just another man who could disappoint. But what she was about to learn is that Jesus wasn't and isn't a man who disappoints. Instead, He loves, cares and provides for. As she began experiencing the love and the acceptance from the people at the Pregnancy Care Center, she began to realize that not all men are like her ex and she started to feel better. She began counseling and learning about all the vitamins she would need to take for her baby to be happy and healthy. As she continued on this journey, she was encouraged to rely on Jesus for His provision and His love and one by one, step by step, she was able to continue her education, she was able to feed, clothe and care for herself and her baby and above all, she began going to Church and reading the Bible to better understand who God is and why He would even want to help her. Today, Norma and Kathy (her daughter) are happy, healthy Christians. Norma is a caregiver for others who find themselves in the same boat and her daughter is excelling at school.

Amazing moments of God's provision.

24

Don't Forget to Thank

I find that this is an excellent point in this book to talk about the power, the goodness, and the appropriateness of giving thanks! We have much thanks to give to God for providing His love directly and through Jesus, to Jesus for His love and perfect sacrifice, and to the Holy Spirit for being our Counselor and Helper through everything. God loves a heart of gratitude and this is something we need to practice each day. We need to thank God for all of the following (and no, this is not an exhaustive or complete list):

His love
His sacrifice
His giving us the earth
His knitting us in our mother's womb
His provision of Jesus and the Holy Spirit
His gift of breath
His gift of nature
His gift of animals
His provision in general
His being there for us each and every step of the way
His continuing to love us even when we have turned our backs on Him or questioned Him
His promises

His creating the Heavens and the earth because they were meant for our good

His teaching us to rely on Him

Him providing us with the opportunities to pray and to let Him know our requests

Him providing us with the opportunities to have and experience visions of goodness He desires to bring into our lives

His providing us with wisdom to intelligently navigate our everyday lives

His provision of family and support

Thanking People

It is also important to give thanks to people. Gratitude is a very powerful concept and tool and used genuinely and authentically, has the power to open many doors. Let's think for a moment about all the people who help each day to make life a little better, a little easier, a little more worth living. Every person from the crossing guards to the teachers to the doctors who help heal people to the authors who take the time to create their written masterpieces to the poets who provide us with great works of art and so much more and so many others.

Each person is there to help you feel better, get from point A to point B, and provide help and services and products that will make our lives better, whether in-person or not.

Do you ever notice when people sit up with their backs' straight or stand tall when they are acknowledged or when their work and/or contribution is acknowledged? They feel good and appreciated and it shows. Why not provide that good praise when a job is well done or a service is well done or even when someone does something kind toward you? Thankfulness is such a powerful tool that we can use to encourage and to show our appreciation and it doesn't even have to cost anything. We can provide that wonderful and appreciated "thank you" to anyone at any time and it makes people feel better. It also actually helps us feel better too because we know that when we provide that, we feel better that we did something kind unto someone else and that we helped that person know that what they did was great and to invite them to keep doing it to us or to someone else.

Praise & Worship

When we thank God for anything, we are providing praise & worship to Him. God loves this and appreciates this act very much. He loves it when His work is acknowledged, He loves when His children praise Him and let Him know that they know the miracle is from Him.

Throughout Scripture, we see God saying "**And you will know that I am the Lord**" (this is said a few times in the Bible including Psalm 46:10). This means that He wants us to know and acknowledge Him and His works in our lives. He wants us to know that these miracles and happenings are from Him and not just random coincidences in our lives. He wants us to realize that He provided for us when nobody else could or would.

It is no error that many Church services begin with praise and with worship. It is not a coincidence that many Pastors fill their sermons with messages and reminders that we are to give Him thanks for all His provisions and to thank Him in advance for the things we would like. It is the same thanks that makes God move and want to do more good works on our behalf. God also loves it when we sing to Him and this is why many services and many Pastors sing a lot either before or during their services and why we have music in Churches.

Lyrics

When we look closely at the lyrics of many songs of worship and praise, we can see that singers and songwriters took the time to painstakingly be inspired and to write out sweet and kind words that convey the Sovereignty of God and do their best to express their love and their worship of God. It is no coincidence that when we hear these songs of praise and worship and we see the lyrics being sung and we can see them plainly on our screens, we can also get choked up and be reminded of God's goodness in our lives and in the lives of those around us.

I am going to use two different songs of worship and provide their lyrics here for you. You may be able to note that the lyrics are entrenched with the singer's love and gratitude to the Lord and how clearly that comes through. If you find a video online of the artist actually singing the song, you will likely notice the passion with which they sing.

I am providing lyrics to songs from two different musicians:

This song is written by Don Moen:

Chorus:
God is good all the time
He put a song of praise in this heart of mine
God is good all the time
Through the darkest night,
His light will shine
God is good, God is good all the time

If you're walking through the valley
And there are shadows all around
Do not fear, He will guide you
He will keep you safe and sound
'Cause He's promised to never leave you
Nor forsake you and His Word is true

Chorus:

God is good all the time
He put a song of praise in this heart of mine
God is good all the time
Through the darkest night, His light will shine
God is good, God is good all the time

We were sinners - so unworthy
Still for us He chose to die
Filled us with His Holy Spirit
Now we can stand and testify
That His love is everlasting
And His mercies - they will never end

Chorus:
God is good all the time
He put a song of praise in this heart of mine
God is good all the time
Through the darkest night, His light will shine
God is good, God is good all the time

Though I may not understand all the plans you have for me,
My life is in your hands
And through the eyes of faith I can clearly see,
Clearly see... God is good.

This next one is written by Elijah Oyelade:

Chorus:
God is good all the time
He put a song of praise in this heart of mine
God is good all the time
Through the darkest night,
His light will shine

God is good, God is good all the time

If you're walking through the valley
And there are shadows all around
Do not fear, He will guide you
He will keep you safe and sound
'Cause He's promised to never leave you
Nor forsake you and His Word is true

Chorus:
God is good all the time
He put a song of praise in this heart of mine
God is good all the time
Through the darkest night, His light will shine
God is good, God is good all the time

We were sinners - so unworthy
Still for us He chose to die
Filled us with His Holy Spirit
Now we can stand and testify
That His love is everlasting
And His mercies - they will never end

Chorus:
God is good all the time
He put a song of praise in this heart of mine
God is good all the time
Through the darkest night, His light will shine
God is good, God is good all the time

Though I may not understand all the plans you have for me,
My life is in your hands
And through the eyes of faith I can clearly see,
Clearly see... God is good.

The Wisdom in Giving Thanks During Difficulties

Some say it is easy to give thanks during the good times - I find it is easier to give thanks during those times too.

But what about during the difficulties? What do we do in terms of thanksgiving during tough times? Do we give thanks for difficulties or do we turn our backs on God at the beginning, middle or end?

I am going to refer to the example of Job here. Job experienced extremely harsh times and extreme difficulties, losing family and his fortune in one swoop. Even his wife told him to curse God and be done with it...but if you read the book of Job, you will know that he did not do that. Did he complain? Yes. Did he question why this was happening? Yes. But did he turn his back on God? No, he didn't. And this is just one reason God counted him as righteous.

Even during the hard times, we must give praise to God because He says in Genesis 50:20 that He will use the evil that was meant to harm us for our benefit. He can turn the situation around with the snap of His fingers and can make things happen that no man can. He can cause the right people to be vindicated and the wrong people to be brought to justice. Many people feel that thanking God and praising Him during a hard time or during hard times is very difficult, and I agree. It is because I have also found it difficult to do that. But I have pushed through and I remember one time when it was really bad, I prayed that He would give me the strength to thank Him and praise Him in that hard time, even though my flesh was dictating otherwise. He did give me that strength and I had to endure the pain for a little while more before He brought me out of it.

Some friends I talked to asked why I chose to praise Him in those difficult times. I reply that **it is because it's in those difficult times that we develop our character, we develop our strength and we develop a**

stronger sense of relying on Him. Some of the best blessings can come out of the most difficult of circumstances and while it stinks while we are going through it and definitely doesn't feel good to our flesh, in the end, we come out stronger and wiser to the ways of the world and how to navigate with wisdom.

In the wise words of Michael Phelps (and I am slightly paraphrasing here): "*Would it really be that great if we always got exactly what we want, exactly when we want it, exactly how we want it? Probably not.*" He is right. It would be great for a little while but then that struggle and that reach for excellence would no longer be there and that struggle and reach for excellence is part of the human condition and the human experience.

Gratitude Journals

One of my very favorite tools is gratitude journals. Gratitude journals are any kind of journal where you write down, jot down, scribble the things you are grateful and thankful for. It can be done by daily entry, as a general blanketed gratitude or it can be done on tablets, construction paper, etc. The purpose of a gratitude journal is to write down and keep a record of the things that make you grateful each day and can include everything from the clean air you breathe, the ability to walk and to smile, the gift of being alive, and more. It can also be gratitude for and to the people in your life, both family and friends. The purpose of the journal (or sheets) is to remember and keep top of mind all the things that mean something to you. I believe gratitude journals and saying thanks should be used every day, without reservation.

It is a wonderful thing for everyone to get into the habit of doing from an early age. Having a family gratitude sharing time can also be a tremendously good and positive use of family time and a great way to remind everyone of the importance of this act. Giving thanks is an act and it is a choice. We can choose to do this or we can not.

I recall some wonderful examples of gratitude journal entries and points I remember seeing over the years from all kinds of people, younger and older. Here are just a few of them:

- Grateful for my mom who goes to work each day to provide for us
- Grateful for my older sister who reads over my school essays
- Thanks to my teacher for teaching us every day, even in a pandemic
- Thanks to the stranger who donated his liver
- Thanks to the person who donated blood to be used during my transfusion
- Thankful to all the frontline care workers (that includes absolutely everyone from doctors and nurses to those who clean the hospitals and more) who worked during the pandemic for our health and wellness
- Thanks to God for providing nature
- Thanks to God for providing His love
- "I want to say thanks to my granpappy for all his love now that he is in heaven"
- Thanks to my friend for always being there and showing me her love
- Thanks to my dad for going to work every day and coming home to still find time and energy to spend with us
- Thanks to the people that brought good food to the food bank so that we had enough to eat when we had no place no live
- Gratitude for the doctor who saved my sister's live during the operation

There are so many more examples, of course. This is a great time to stop and at this point in the book, give you a chance to write out your gratitude list. Remember that it isn't about how many things you write, it is about its meaning in your life. If you would like, write down next to it why it is so meaningful to you. As an added little step: you can also create your own little paper mache or other artistic design gratitude booklet that you design yourself and you can enjoy looking at, reading your entries and adding to it over the years as you continue in your life steps. Here is some space to get started:

Giving Thanks in the Bible

I want to share some of the Biblical verses on giving thanks and where they are found in the Bible. I believe these will help remind you of how Biblical giving thanks really is, in addition to giving you the references so you can go and read more about the context in the given book.

- "Give thanks to the Lord, for he is good; his love endures forever." 1 Chronicles 16:34
- "Let the peace of Christ rule in your hearts, since as members of one body you were called to peace. And be thankful." Colossians 3:15
- "Devote yourselves to prayer, being watchful and thankful." Colossians 4:2
- "I always thank my God for you because of his grace given you in Christ Jesus." 1 Corinthians 1:4
- "You will be enriched in every way so that you can be generous on every occasion, and through us your generosity will result in thanksgiving to God." 2 Corinthians 9:11
- "For everything God created is good, and nothing is to be rejected if it is received with thanksgiving, because it is consecrated by the word of God and prayer." 1 Timothy 4:4-5
- "Rejoice always, pray continually, give thanks in all circumstances; for this is God's will for you in Christ Jesus." 1 Thessalonians 5:16-18
- "Do not be anxious about anything, but in every situation, by prayer and petition, with thanksgiving, present your requests to God. And the peace of God, which transcends all understanding, will guard your hearts and your minds in Christ Jesus." Philippians 4:6-7
- "But I, with shouts of grateful praise, will sacrifice to you. What I have vowed I will make good. I will say, 'Salvation comes from the Lord.'" Jonah 2:9
- "The Lord is my strength and my shield; in him my heart trusts, and I am helped; my heart exults, and with my song I give thanks to him." Psalm 28:7

- "Offer to God a sacrifice of thanksgiving, and perform your vows to the Most High." Psalm 50:14
- "You have put more joy in my heart than they have when their grain and wine abound." Psalm 4:7
- "Surely he says this for us, doesn't he? Yes, this was written for us, because when farmers plow and thresh, they should be able to do so in the hope of sharing in the harvest." 1 Corinthians 9:10
- "Now he who supplies seed to the sower and bread for food will also supply and increase your store of seed and will enlarge the harvest of your righteousness." 2 Corinthians 9:10
- "Let us not become weary in doing good, for at the proper time we will reap a harvest if we do not give up." Galatians 6:9
- "You have enlarged the nation and increased their joy; they rejoice before you as people rejoice at the harvest, as soldiers rejoice when dividing the plunder." Isaiah 9:3
- "They do not say to themselves, 'Let us fear the Lord our God, who gives autumn and spring rains in season, who assures us of the regular weeks of harvest.'" Jeremiah 5:24
- "The earth has yielded its produce; God, our God, blesses us." Psalm 67:6
- "From the fruit of their mouths people's stomachs are filled; with the harvest of their lips they are satisfied." Proverbs 18:20
- "Then another angel came out of the temple and called in a loud voice to him who was sitting on the cloud, 'Take your sickle and reap, because the time to reap has come, for the harvest of the earth is ripe.'" Revelation 14:15
- "Let the word of Christ dwell in you richly, teaching and admonishing one another in all wisdom, singing psalms and hymns and spiritual songs, with thankfulness in your hearts to God." Colossians 3:16
- "Therefore, since we are receiving a kingdom that cannot be shaken, let us be thankful, and so worship God acceptably with reverence and awe, for our 'God is a consuming fire.'" Hebrews 12:28-29

- "Sing to the Lord, all the earth; proclaim his salvation day after day. Declare his glory among the nations, his marvelous deeds among all peoples. For great is the Lord and most worthy of praise; he is to be feared above all gods. For all the gods of the nations are idols, but the Lord made the heavens." 1 Chronicles 16:23-26
- "And now we thank you, our God, and praise your glorious name." 1 Chronicles 29:13
- "Through him then let us continually offer up a sacrifice of praise to God, that is, the fruit of lips that acknowledge his name." Hebrews 13:15
- "The Lord is my strength and my shield; my heart trusts in him, and he helps me. My heart leaps for joy, and with my song I praise him. Psalm 28:7
- "In God, whose word I praise—in God I trust and am not afraid. What can mere mortals do to me?" Psalm 56:4
- "I will praise the name of God with a song; I will magnify him with thanksgiving." Psalm 69:30
- "I will sing of the Lord's great love forever; with my mouth I will make your faithfulness known through all generations. I will declare that your love stands firm forever, that you have established your faithfulness in heaven itself." Psalm 89:1-2
- "Oh come, let us sing to the Lord; let us make a joyful noise to the rock of our salvation! Let us come into his presence with thanksgiving; let us make a joyful noise to him with songs of praise! For the Lord is a great God, and a great King above all gods." Psalm 95:1-3
- "It is good to praise the Lord and make music to your name, O Most High, proclaiming your love in the morning and your faithfulness at night, to the music of the ten-stringed lyre and the melody of the harp." Psalm 92:1-3
- "Enter his gates with thanksgiving and his courts with praise; give thanks to him and praise his name." Psalm 100:4
- "Let them give thanks to the Lord for his unfailing love and his

wonderful deeds for mankind, for he satisfies the thirsty and fills the hungry with good things." Psalm 107:8-9
- "Finally, brothers and sisters, whatever is true, whatever is noble, whatever is right, whatever is pure, whatever is lovely, whatever is admirable—if anything is excellent or praiseworthy—think about such things." Philippians 4:8
- "Rejoice always, pray without ceasing, give thanks in all circumstances; for this is the will of God in Christ Jesus for you." 1 Thessalonians 5:16-18

As part of your daily practice, try to give thanks a few times in your day and give yourself helpful reminders to do so. Most people (if not all) really appreciate this and will remember the person that gave them thanks and how it made them feel.

Giving thanks is also a way to show and extend grace because we don't have to give thanks, we are choosing to do so.

25

Spend Time in the Word....On Purpose

One of the smartest things you can do in your day is to spend time reading the Bible. If possible, take some time each morning to spend time in the Word, asking the Holy Spirit to outline for you and to bring things to your attention that you need to know about and work on, as well as things you already do well.

One of the very best ways to get to know God, Jesus and the Holy Spirit is to spend time in the Word and to get to see and experience the stories, experiences and encounters of others who came before you. The old adage of learning from the errors of others is true and we would be wise to try to not repeat the same mistakes others before us have made. **Remember that we now have the advantage of reading and knowing about those stories, which means that we are in a better place (better equipped) to do better, now that we have watched the good works and the errors of others.**

> **An amazing thing happens when we spend time reading God's Word: we feel peace.**

An amazing thing happens when we spend time in the Word: we feel peace. We become much more peaceful when we read the Bible. I have had this experience many times and it's almost like a blanket of peace comes over you as you read the Bible and you see God's provision for those who came before us. It is also pretty cool to see the supernatural wonders (hello burning bush, hello parting of the Red Sea, hello a virgin getting pregnant, hello turning water into wine, hello Jesus walking on water, hello a staff becoming a serpent, hello prison door locks falling off, hello men being rescued from the furnace that has been turned up ten times hotter, and many, many more examples).

When we read about these supernatural happenings, we are informed (for some) and reminded (for others) of the power of God and how He can make things happen. It's like you go through your day remembering these things and knowing that "God's got you!"

Activating the Holy Spirit

I know I said this further up but it is so important, it bears repeating. Before we read the Bible, even before we pray, it would be wise to pray for the Holy Spirit to open the eyes of our heart and to illuminate passages, and stories that we need to pay particular attention to. If you are anything like me in my early years of my Christian walk, I would read the Bible and understand nothing. I am not exaggerating - I understood nothing. It is then that my Godfather, Berj Basmadjian, gifted me with a student Bible. This was such an easy, simple way for me to understand the Bible, its teachings and to begin to understand this wonderful book. Without this student Bible to start and the opportunity to see student notes explaining Biblical concepts, I would have stayed lost.

As of this writing, I had spent some time just yesterday talking to a gentleman to whom I was ministering and he said to me that he understood nothing when he read the Bible. This is not an uncommon feeling and sentiment. Many people don't and so having versions like that, that can simplify and break things down for us (at least until we get to a later point where we can understand more easily and we can move on to the regular Bible) is extremely helpful. It's not that people are not smart enough to understand it when they are reading it, it's that it contains so many new names, new terms, new phenomena that it is very easy to get a little bit overwhelmed or we may not understand or interpret things completely.

Another thing we can do to better understand is to pray to the Holy Spirit for a better understanding of the Bible's contents. Here is a suggested prayer you can use to this end. Remember that you can always pray in your mind (God can hear your thoughts) or you can pray out loud.:

"Lord Jesus, I know how much wisdom is available in the Bible and as You know, I am finding it challenging in some ways to understand its content. I pray for the Holy Spirit to talk to me, to enlighten me, to bring an understanding of the stories, events, characters and more in the Bible so that I may gain an understanding. I pray for the Holy Spirit to really speak to me very clearly and to help me understand all that I am reading and to really be able to relate the stories to my life. In Jesus' name. Amen."

Bible Apps

With the more widespread use of technology, we have the benefit of being able to download and use Bible apps totally free of charge, to undertake mini courses of study to help us better understand the Bible and to apply its teachings to our lives, to highlight and keep track of key passages, and more!

Even if you want a hard copy for yourself, there are many Christian organizations that provide copies free of charge. You can simply go to the organization's website, put in your information or call them and they will mail you a copy.

> **You can get the wisest book written, directly inspired by God and teaches you all about life's lessons, rules and principles given to you free of charge. Sounds like a pretty good deal to me!**

Why I Say "On Purpose" in the Chapter Title

We all get busy and we all have many things vying for our attention and response. We have children and family life, bills, we have chores and homework, we have places to go and visit and people to meet and see, etc. People have many things to do and those things can sometimes (or often) prevent us from sitting in quiet and spending time in the Word. Being busy can be really good, but if you are so busy that you do not have time to spend a few minutes during your morning or when you need it in your day, this means that you are too busy. That too is a strategy of the enemy: to keep you so busy that you don't have time to spend in the Word, weakening your faith and not allowing you time to pray, reflect, meditate and spend time talking to and listening to God.

I remember very clearly how a friend of mine resolved to spend time in the Word each morning (or at least at some point in her day) and she declared this to me out loud over the phone one Sunday. She had mentioned that she was feeling disconnected and felt that it was important to get back to that connection and enjoy her time with the Lord. What happened next was very interesting. She recounted how starting from the moment when she had said that, all craziness broke loose: she got messages, phone calls, work emails and much, much more, including new and unexpected bills and expenses that she hadn't prepared for. She told me at the end of the day on Tuesday that since the moment she said that to me on Sunday night, that everything went nuts and that she had spent zero time in the Word since she had that and with no end in sight to her obligations, guaranteeing that she would be further prevented from spending that much-needed time. I suggested she pray about it and ask God to lift the unnecessary burdens so that she could follow through on her promise and once she did that, things started to settle down.

So if you can find even 15 minutes in your morning to spend that time, it is worth it because those 15 minutes can carry you through your entire day.

Praying & Reading in Your Car or in Transit

We may be at an appointment, waiting to be seen, waiting for our kid's activity to be done and so we may have a few minutes, or we may be in line somewhere, waiting our turn to be seen or served. Regardless of where it is or when, you can find a few minutes in your car or in transit to read, to pray, to do a devotional, to type your gratitude into your smartphone notes, etc. I can't tell you how many times I have prayed while I was in my car driving from point A to point B on a particularly busy day.

On busy days, I have also prayed that God would provide perfect timing so that I could get everything that I needed to do done and in good time. Each time I had prayed this, the timing of things worked out beautifully.

Praying Away the Unimportant

Sometimes, we may be doing something that we think is important but in later reflection, we see that it actually was not. Again, the enemy is good at causing us to be busy with the unimportant so that we get too busy and don't spend time on the important. For example, a parent who has started a business that would take them away from spending quality time with their kids but they didn't ask God if starting that business was His will for them. They could easily be thinking that this is something else I need to do, but it may not be the case, and what it did was to pull your time and attention away from things that needed and required more of you, making you unable to do "all of it" and then causing you to feel bad and feel mediocre. Before you undertake something, big or small, ask God about it. Ask Him if the idea is from Him.

I remember long ago when I was just starting my Christian walk, I woke up with the idea to write a book on a certain topic. I started to get excited about it and started to think about when I could use time in my day to write this book. I shared the idea with my Christian friend who had been the one talking to me about a relationship with Christ and she asked me some probing questions about the book, its topic and scope. As I began and continued describing it, she said (in a loving and supportive way), "*Chris, I don't think this is the right thing to do. I don't think this book idea is from God.*" I was a bit perplexed by her response but I said that I would take time to think about it and pray about it. And I did. I began to realize that the idea for the book had nothing to do with God and certainly was not an idea that would honor Him in any way. I saw how an idea had been dropped into my mind - one that would take me away from spending the very much-needed quality time with God and that would have taken me away from reading my newly-acquired student Bible.

Years later and now in hindsight, I made the right decision to not write that book. We need to be mindful of where and how we are spending our time.

Hanging Up Stickies

When we are reading the Word, and especially when a passage or a phrase jumps out at us, we would be wise to write it down on a piece of paper, or on a card and hang it up. It is helpful to have Bible verses and quotes hung up around the house, so that we can be reminded of them and continue mulling them over in our subconscious as we go through our day. This is something I did when I was living on my own and I found it a tremendous help to me because it allowed me to let the passage or phrase really sit and settle in my mind, consciously and subconsciously, and allowed me to keep it top of mind no matter what else I was doing in my day.

Also, when you are reading a Bible passage and it leaps out to you, this is the Holy Spirit trying to tell you something that you need to know about it. It could be related to something you are dealing with or will be dealing with. Either way, you can pray to know why this particular passage leaped out to you in terms of its relevance in your life.

Love Yourself & Accept God's Love....On the Bathroom Mirror

We all sometimes struggle with loving and appreciating ourselves. We all sometimes struggle with reminding ourselves how wonderful we are and how much Jesus loves us despite our sin, our imperfections and our wrong ways. We can all use that extra happy jolt of reminding ourselves how loved and how lucky we are. One way to do that is to have little notes or stickies on the bathroom mirror, the dresser, our kitchen cabinets, etc., that remind us of this love. Especially on those days when we feel unlovable and we may feel undesirable, these little notes can go a long way to keep your spirits up and to remind you of how much God loves you.

Some examples of these notes could be:

- God loves me
- Jesus loves me
- God cherishes me
- Jesus thought I was to die for
- God thinks I am precious
- I have been so blessed and am grateful to be so
- God's love wraps me up each and every day
- God loved me even before He knitted me in my mother's stomach
- God gave me the skills and talents of _____. I am awesome
- I love me because God loved me first

These stickies and notes are a great, life-affirming way of keeping God top of mind and helping to build ourselves up. There are more than enough things in the world trying to tear us down, so let's use this as one tool to build ourselves back up.

You can do this for yourself and it's always nice and appreciated to do it for others, too. Write your spouse or your kids or your parents or your sibling a little note or many notes, telling them you appreciate their good qualities, how you noted that they did something for you, how you encourage them and more. Putting this somewhere where they may not expect it would be such a welcome surprise to them. For example, if your spouse makes you coffee each morning, you can put a little note on the coffee maker he or she uses to thank them for being so thoughtful and making you your coffee every day.

Imagine how good and how built-up you and your family members or whomever you live with would feel if you got into a daily practice of doing this. It may feel a bit weird at first but you will get used to it and you and everyone doing it will reap the tremendous benefits of it.

If you are a parent or a guardian, think about how much it would positively impact your children to spend time each day or each week building each other up with God's Word and spending time reading the Word each day would be for their own walk. Children will usually value and continue practicing those things their parent(s) or guardian(s) value and that they watched these acts taking place as they were growing up.

> It may even be a really nice idea to include a weekly schedule where Bible reading and study time are included and featured, as would be something I refer to as "happy time", which is the time we remind ourselves in a humble way how wonderful we are and how much God loves us.

These wonderful items are great things to include in your schedules because they benefit everyone and in this day-and-age where young and old are experiencing mental health issues (or even crises), they would benefit everyone tremendously by providing foundational tools on which to build self-esteem and self-love, among the many other solid values presented in the Bible.

26

Pay It Forward

When something good and fortunate happens for you or to you, thank God and pay it forward. Paying it forward means that you don't pay back in kindness or in favor of the person who was good to you but instead, you provide a kindness or goodness to another person.

For example, a former coworker of mine helped me out a lot one day of a very bad snow blizzard by shoveling the snow around my car to clear the pathway for me to get out and cleaned the snow off my car. When I got to the parking lot after work, I was expecting to find my little car covered in snow and expected that it would be very hard to dig my way out and I expected to be outside in the cold, cleaning off my car and having to figure out a way to plow my car out of the driveway and onto the street. Instead, I got to my car and found that she had cleaned off my car and plowed the area around me. She was still in the parking lot doing this same work for others and when I thanked her for her kindness, she asked me to simply "pay it forward". I did and helped an elderly man at the gas station I later went to.

Such kindnesses are never really forgotten and are always appreciated.

When we take the time to be good to others, to do someone a favor, to extend our kindness and thoughtfulness to a person, amazing things happen. Both people feel good, the world becomes just a bit of a better place and it can cause many more good actions and good results can come from those first ones. It is a chain effect and it only has to stop, well, never. We can keep doing wonderful things for others and with no expectation that we will ever get anything out of it, but the way God works is that we will get plenty out of it each time.

I was driving in the car one day and I heard on the radio about a mechanic who was volunteering his time to fix up old cars in his free time and gifts them to rural families without a ride. Eliot Middleton is a barbecue restaurant owner and a trained mechanic in South Carolina who has decided to perform this service free of charge. You may be asking where did he (or does he) get the money for the parts and Middleton explained that people began donating the parts so that he could accomplish his task of fixing up the car. Further, it has been widely reported that people all around the country offered to donate almost 800 cars and more than $100,000 in cash as well. What Middleton is doing is amazing and he is not asking for anything to do this. He is paying it forward and has also become an outlet to allow others to pay it forward through him as well. This would be a great opportunity to think about how you too can pay it forward. Remember that paying it forward does not have to be only financial payment.

27

Tithing

Tithing is an ancient Biblical concept of paying to God the first 10% of our income so that God can use that money to bless others and can pay you back manifold.

The Scripture for this is found in Malachi 3:10 "**Bring the whole tithe into the storehouse, that there may be food in my house. Test me in this,**" says the Lord Almighty "**and see if I will not throw open the floodgates of heaven and pour out so much blessing that you will not have room enough for it...**" Now, paying tithes and giving the money to God does not mean literally giving Him the money. No. We tithe by financially supporting organizations that reflect the values and the goodness of Jesus, such as Churches and charities that honor and value Jesus. Unfortunately not every place that touts that it is a Church is one that follows and adheres to the Bible. Some say that they do but when you look deeply at their value statements and practices, you can see that they do not uphold Jesus' values.

Also, soup kitchens, homeless shelters, and other beautiful charities that recognize and uphold the values of Jesus and the Word are the ones I choose to provide my tithes payments to. In order to not be misled and to give your tithes to a worthwhile organization, we need to pray about the place and see what God tells us about it. For example,

I prayed about a Church I was considering tithing to and asked God about whether I should give them my tithes or somewhere else. He told me in no uncertain terms that this Church was not following correct practices and that they were doing many wrong things. I was shocked because I assumed that they were doing the right thing. Not so. So, I decided to give my tithes to another Christian organization that the Lord guided me to.

It is not enough for an organization to be doing good things. That's lovely but we are looking specifically for organizations that recognize, love, honor and follow Christ in their daily practices.

Not Just An Ancient Custom

I should also mention here that many people I have spoken to over the years think that this is an ancient custom, and not one that God asks or expects us to use today. That is not true. Tithing is as relevant today as it was back then and we need to remember the Lord each time we incur income and then watch as He multiplies it. According to my experiences and the experiences of others around me, He multiplies this money in various amazing ways and He always provides. Now, please note that the process does not work like clockwork, in that you don't pay tithes and then, BING, you get that money five-fold or ten-fold back into your wallet or your bank account. It simply doesn't work that way. The process (I have come to learn is as follows):

1. Knowledge that you need to pay your tithes.
2. Choosing to comply and to pay your tithes.
3. Praying about the right, Christ-centered organization to which to make the payment.
4. Pay your tithes and ensure the organization has received it.
5. Wait in faith.
6. Receive your own blessing.

The process of receiving does not come instantly. You have to wait for it and you have to stay in faith that He is bringing it. Many people choose to give up during the wait period and I would advise against that.

Having said all of that, our reason for tithing cannot and should not be that we want to receive money back. Our reason for tithing needs to be that we want and desire to see the advancement of the Kingdom of Heaven and God's good works. God knows and sees your heart so He knows your true intentions and motives. If you are unsure about your own motives, pray and ask God to reveal to you what He knows to be true about you. It is a great and important way to "get right" with Him on this very important topic.

God Wants Us To Be Rich

I covered this earlier in another chapter but I find it so important to mention this again that I will use this little section here to talk about this again for a moment. God does want us to be rich and this may come as a shock to some but He wants us to have great health and great wealth.

I was having this conversation with a Christian lady (or at least, she calls herself a Christian lady) and she tried to challenge me on this point, almost to the point of scoffing, and saying outright that that is not true. I pointed out Biblical examples to prove this but she wasn't having any of it. Biblically, the Lord instructs us to have a peaceful and respectful conversation but then if the other person chooses not to believe or not to engage, then we are to leave it alone. After I tried respectfully and with Biblical support to make my point, and I could see she was not receiving it, I decided to leave it alone. You cannot make people do anything and if that's the value she sees as fit, then I let God deal with her in the ways He knows how.

So do go to whatever work you do, make money, invest your money and hopefully you will see it grow and you will prosper. All riches are available to us who believe and as long as we are working on attaining these riches in the right ways, and checking with Him to make sure that our ways are correct, then we know that we are doing right and we can go in peace.

Testimonials of Tithing

I know how helpful it is to see evidence of things having worked for others. This is an important thing to experience and I know I used to look for it when I was considering tithing for the first time. So, I checked out a few different Christian organizations like the 700 Club who used to talk about and outline tithing testimonials. People who had tithed talked a lot about how they gave in faith and the financial and abundant miracles they experienced after they patiently and in faith waited following their donation or their gift. It isn't easy to step out in faith but you can trust God and what He says. You can believe in Him and see how it happened for so many others before you.

I remember watching story after story of people who gave money in faith and in obedience (and cheerfully so) and how they were so blessed in all different ways. Another great thing about actually tithing is the joy, happiness and warmth you get when you give money for a cause and to people who are in need and you help to support them through the goodness that Jesus has provided you.

I invite you to check out testimonials if you are so inclined and to step out in faith and to tithe as you feel led to do.

Being....and Remaining.....Humble

Success is also about being humble. We are equipped to do the most wonderful works and many do, but if we don't remain humble, then we lose sight of what's most important.

People learn best from those who have faith, work hard and don't get ahead of themselves. There is nothing wrong with being pleased with our accomplishments (there was a full chapter earlier in this book about just that) but we need to learn to praise Jesus and to thank Him for what He has done, not what we have done. According to Phillipians 4:13, 14, we "can do all things through Christ who strengthens us" and we know that it is the Holy Spirit that lights our way so **when the breakthrough happens and we accomplish what we need to, we need to give credit to God. He is the beginning and end of our faith. He is the way, the truth and the life. One of the best things to say when we have accomplished something is to say "praise Jesus."**

Also, when we accomplish something, it is fitting to help others who come after us. Others need that support, that leg up, that help just as much as you did before your success. Not providing that is not being humble but instead, being prideful. For instance, I am reminded of a case where a woman had made a fantastic film that was the toast of the town (I loved it too) and she had really done a great job. The movie was fun, colorful, snappy, cute, and had a fantastic script. I was in LA listening to her talking about her beginnings and how she thought of putting the whole project together. Then, at the end of the interview, a sweet and earnest young girl who had been in the audience asked her if she would help her in any way, if she would mentor her, if she would give her any opportunities for her to learn with her. The filmmaker's answer was no. She was not going to provide her with that opportunity. I think this young girl would have appreciated any help, and I don't think her intention was to take up too much of her time or to be troublesome, just to get some help. I could see how the girl was crushed when she got the response and it's not something I will forget. The filmmaker had a chance to help and to be humble and to pay it forward and she did not take it.

Another example that I felt was less-than-exemplary is a real estate agent who boasted his stats on social media. He had a big post congratulating himself on having made millions in a relatively short amount of time and while others may have looked at it in awe, I found it to be distasteful. It is great that you are doing very well in your career, but boasting about it in that way is neither appealing nor is it appropriate.

Being An Example

When we are successful and humble, we begin to become an example to others. Being successful, humble and wanting to help others are qualities that I think are the marks of true leaders, of true success stories. Just because a person has the biggest home, the fanciest car and material possessions, it doesn't mean they can't also be humble and the reverse is true too.

In the action-packed thriller movie, Red Notice, Ryan Reynolds plays a humorous character who, while he is amazing at his action-packed stunts and his quick-thinking moves, he is also humble and hilariously self-deprecating. He keeps things happy and light in the movie with his antics, his one-liners and his offbeat, very charming personality. He is a star in the field of movies that never seems to take himself too seriously and that seems to always put the every man ahead of himself.

I also watched another film star, Dwayne "The Rock" Johnson take an opportunity for giving. He gifted a veteran his own personal truck and did so just to demonstrate kindness. Please read the story here (taken from Vulture.com):

Dwayne "The Giving" Johnson invited fans to a special screening of his Netflix film *Red Notice* and wanted to make the day extra special for them. He originally wanted to give away the Porsche Taycan he drives in the movie but was unsuccessful. However, The Rock had a bigger idea: to give away his favorite custom truck. He was especially moved by one fan named Oscar's story: he was a navy veteran, personal trainer, church leader, and volunteer at a domestic violence center. Johnson invited Oscar on the stage, thanked him for what he did for the community, and then took him outside to surprise him with his new car. Once reading the card that declared the custom truck to be his, Oscar fell to the ground in gratitude and thanked Johnson. He then called his girlfriend to show her his new friend and his new ride. Hopefully, Johnson can continue to surprise fans by appearing in *Fast 10*.

When a movie star or any man demonstrates that kind of forward-thinking, thoughtfulness, kindness and that kind of humbleness, it is infectious, emotion-inducing and it promotes the concept of humbleness and giving in the minds of others. What a fantastic example that will be read by millions!

One other example comes to mind. Kawhi Leonard is one of the great basketball legends of our time. When you realize how hard he works despite his tremendous talent, it is amazing to see. He is also noted as one of the kindest people around. Here is a bit about him, taken from BleacherReport.com:

Leonard personifies the humble and quiet star who internalizes nearly all his emotions and just outworks everyone, despite his enormous talent.
Many people questioned whether Leonard would ever be good enough to warrant the cost of trading away Hill, so he went to work proving doubters wrong.
He has improved his scoring, blocks and assists every year since he

joined the league in 2011, and he broke through in the 2014 NBA Finals when the Spurs won the championship and Leonard earned MVP honors at the tender age of 22.

"When Kawhi makes a mistake, he's almost apologetic. He doesn't want to disappoint anybody. There are times he does something well, and I have to tell him, 'That was super. That was fantastic. That was a helluva job. You can smile now. You can feel great about yourself.'"

Humility, hard work and a constant hustling ethic make Leonard not only a top-five player, but also one of the most admired superstars in the NBA.

These are two men that many people (especially young people) look up to. They do good unto others and they work very hard, in addition to having innate talent. These are wonderful examples for young people everywhere to work hard, stay humble (have humility) and to put your best into all you do. They also teach that when we make a mistake, we need to apologize and call it our bad. People can fault you for having made a mistake (we all make them) but they cannot fault you for taking ownership of those mistakes and stepping up to do whatever you can do to rectify those mistakes.

People who do these things have the genuine marks of leadership and of humility and humbleness and prove to be wonderful examples to all those who are lucky enough to have seen, heard or witnessed their goodness in some way.

My last example in this section is of a guy named Dave. Many years ago, we were having a barbecue at work and a few people were taking turns on the grill. The BBQ was meant to be for the students at the school and the staff. Each person was allowed to take one burger and sides of their choice. The burgers were being handed out and people started to devour them (they were really good). I had asked Dave if he was going to help himself to a burger, as everyone else was and he said he would not. He said that he hadn't yet done anything to help with the BBQ (he had been in class teaching) so he promptly made his way outside to help with the BBQ. He relieved the staff member who was at the grill and was surely exhausted and he started grilling burgers for everyone else. It was only after he had exhausted himself and he had contributed significantly to the BBQ that he allowed himself to have a burger. Why do I mention this? Because he humbly would not partake in the enjoyment of the food without having contributed something. That is being a person of integrity and to really putting your best into what you do. Further, as a teacher, he knew students would be looking and watching, taking example and having seen that he believed he needed to work for his reward. He provided a solid example of humble service as he wouldn't partake in the food and satisfy his hunger unless he had first helped significantly. A truly noble and humble attitude!

28

Christ-Based Marriages & Family Life

Readers, Biblical marriages are meant to include three entities: husband, wife and Jesus.

When we take Jesus out of the equation, we are setting ourselves up for a particularly hard time in our marriage. Everyone goes through trials in their marriage, everyone goes through difficulties, everyone goes through hardships (no matter how strong a couple you are) but Jesus is there to help you both through those difficulties. Ladies, you may be feeling angry or frustrated that your husband is working long and late hours, and you may have all kinds of ideas going through your mind. Or husbands, your wife could be out with some friends and you start to get ideas in your mind of what could be going on. These are normal thoughts to have but we don't have to stick to those thoughts. We don't have to keep those thoughts active. We can choose to dismiss them or if you feel worried, pray about them. You can and should ask the Holy Spirit to speak to you about what you are feeling and whether there is legitimacy to what you are feeling.

Sometimes, spouses can become prideful and they don't want to admit to their spouse, to friends, to family or even to themselves that they may be feeling insecure, not sure their spouse is still committed to them or as committed to them as they used to be, not sure they are still attractive to their spouse or a myriad of other worries that can come. When we let these thoughts fester, when we don't pray through them, when we let worries, anxieties and fears build up and we don't take the time to talk to our spouse about them, we can create a disconnect in our relationship and your spouse may be feeling hurt that you don't care, may be feeling distant from you or a whole host of other destructive thoughts running through your mind or his. We have to talk to our spouse, we have to share, we have to live out the values in Scripture in our marriage. We have to cherish our spouse and treat them like they are the fine treasures that we know they are.

> **Our role as a spouse is to cherish our husband or wife, to treat them like the masterpiece that they are, and to remember how blessed we are to be married to them. That is the promise we made on our wedding day.**

There will inevitably be times where you feel exhausted, where you feel stretched and where you may even be feeling like you're at the end of your rope. This may very well happen often too and that's ok because those are the times to go to Jesus in prayer and admit that you feel lost, worried, scared, alone, abandoned, hurt, whatever. He is there to talk to you and He will guide you to talk to your spouse where and when the time is right. Just talking to our spouses can often be the case that helps to mend everything and sometimes, it's putting aside our own desires and realizing that maybe you are trying to go down a path that you are not meant to.

For example, I was ministering to a man one time who said that his girlfriend wanted to engage in some physical activities that he wasn't comfortable with. He enjoyed kissing and being physical in those senses, but he didn't feel comfortable going further. When I asked him why, he said he didn't know but that he also didn't want his girlfriend to think he was "a wimp". After further ministering to him and trying to understand why he didn't feel right about going further, I pointed out that he was actually exemplifying and embodying Biblical values because he wanted to wait until they were married and that he should be pleased with himself for honoring them both in that way. He realized that his hesitancy was based on the fact that in his heart or hearts, he felt that it was wrong to take things further without the covenant of marriage binding them. When he spoke to his girlfriend about it, she was neither empathetic nor was she understanding about his feelings, which is not fair, kind or respectful. He made the decision to end the relationship and to pray for God to bring him a woman who would embody and exemplify the same values he believed were important.

Suzanne and Jack were a young couple who had been set up by a friend. They had been dating for 3 years. Suzanne knew she was in love with Jack and wanted a future with him and Jack seemed into her but seemed to be taking his time and being quite non-committal. He suggested they begin looking for a home together but Suzanne felt confused because she had made it clear that she wanted to at least be engaged before looking for a home together. Even the friend who set them up was confused about why Jack was dragging his feet. When they gently asked him about it, he gave a very vague, non-committal answer and refused to take things to the next level. He insisted that he only wanted to move in together and keep things that way, something Suzanne and her family were not in approval of. In the end, Jack decided not to move things forward and broke things off, perplexing Suzanne and the friend who set them up. Today, Jack is single and each time he revisits his lack of making the move to engagements, he speaks of regret but does not move things forward to do anything about it.

Pray For Your Spouse & Kids

Just about every person on planet earth who has a spouse and, or has children worries about them. This is part of human nature. We cannot be everywhere at once and try as we may, we cannot always be physically there with our loved ones. No, we need to rely instead on God to watch over them, protect them, be with them. But many forget one important part that is needed to activate God watching over their families: praying for that. Many people forget to pray for the protection of their loved ones and only begin to do so when trouble has already made its way over to them. Praying each day a little prayer for the protection of your loved ones is not overdoing it and letting your family know that you are praying for them causes them to appreciate you, to cherish what you are doing for them and ultimately, brings you all closer.

A young man I taught one time had begun to harm himself, and I discovered it. When I spoke to the other staff members about it, they advised me to talk to the appropriate staff member. I did that and a little while later, it was revealed that this young man had been hurting himself for weeks because his parents were going through a very difficult time, causing him and his little brother to think that their parents didn't love them anymore. When his parents heard this, they let him and his little brother know that they loved them very much and that they would be attending counseling sessions to help their marriage, helping both boys feel better. At the end of the session, though, came a very nice moment: the parents told the kids that even though they had been arguing a lot, they hoped and prayed for the well-being of the boys, and they didn't want them to harm themselves in any way. This was an incredibly touching moment for the family, one that I hope will guide them onto a much healthier path.

Praying for all members of our family is not a frill - it's something we need to do each day and each day they come home, we need to thank

God for keeping them safe. Friends, we are living in difficult times when all members of the family are going through a lot and not only do families need to pull together, spend time in Scripture together and work together for the best of everyone in the family, but younger children need to be taught about the love Jesus has for them, and all the goodness that is available in Him.

Some parents don't know the good that is available in Christ and so I encourage you to pick up your Bible, to attend Bible study classes, attend Bible-based Church services, be part of your local Churches, whatever you can do to get your family into the Word of God.

I will provide another example. I have a dear friend I will call Sheila. I knew her marriage was not a healthy one and that things were not going well in general with her family. I knew that her husband drank and I knew that she felt like the whole world was sitting on her shoulders. I knew that she needed her husband's support but that he was simply not available. I also learned that he had come home drunk one night and hit one of his sons, something that his daughter saw and admitted later that it traumatized her. Sheila was doing her best at keeping everything together and she was doing her best at maintaining a happy(ish) home and family life but things were coming apart at the seams. I will never forget when she finally opened up to me about their financial, home and marital situation and how dire things had become and how the children's welfare agencies were involved. I mentioned and advised her to get resources and some help from a few different places in an effort to quench all that had been going on and while she was doing all that was needed, he had made the decision to cut his ties and to move away from the family. Today, Sheila and her children are in a good Bible-based Church but her ex-husband continues to spiral.

You Are Both Invited To Get Into The Word & Read Devotionals

Having a healthy, Christ-centered marriage necessarily requires both members spending time in the Word, getting their minds renewed and remembering to cherish their spouse each day. Spending time in the Word and reading devotionals separately and together allows you both to set aside time for each other, to connect or to reconnect, to rekindle that special time, and to use that time to strengthen your marriage. You will find yourselves being much stronger heads of the family when you are strong in your marriage, when you feel connected with your spouse and when you take time to cherish each other.

Watching Mom and Dad

Kids, tweens, teens and young adults are always watching their parents or their guardians. They are watching, listening and learning to see how they treat each other, how they interact and if they take the time to honor Christ and each other. This is the foundation of their development as children and no matter how old they get, it will cause an indelible imprint on them and will affect them going forward.

One young man was very mean in speaking to his wife despite the fact that he said he loved her. When they went to counseling together, he was trying to understand why he would speak so harshly with his wife. The counselor wisely asked about his upbringing and when he reflected and then pointed out that he had grown up watching and hearing his parents fight and argue, and his dad berating his mother constantly, it severely left a negative impression on him and he felt that that was the only right way to deal with your spouse. It took a bit of counseling for him to realize that he was repeating a negative and destructive pattern of behavior that he had grown up with and that he had to consciously stop doing this in order to see his marriage survive and thrive, and for his children to have a positive example in their home life.

Achievements

No matter their age, children have a much greater chance at high levels of achievements when they grow up with solid family values: eating right, getting the right amount of sleep, finishing your homework, spending quality family time, sharing and supporting each other and having a good time and laughing together and, last but not least, enjoying time in the Word. Children who grow up with these solid family values, tweens and teens who continue to have these solid family values, even young adults and adults who see excellent values in the home have much greater chances of doing well. These are the same values they will then take into their own future home life when they are old enough and have their own family.

I used to watch students speak so negatively: "I suck at this" "I'm totally going to fail this test, I'm such an idiot" "I studied but I'm so dumb, I'll never get this". I had to ask the students to consciously stop speaking this over their lives and to speak positively, using phrases like **"I've got this!" "I know I can do this" "I studied and I'm going to put my best into what I'm doing"** and **"I may not know everything but I sure know a lot and I feel I'm going to do great because I'm going to put my best into this."**

When we teach kids, tweens, teens, and young adults to speak positively, they begin to feel better about themselves, and they begin to see themselves in a more positive way. They don't have to already be a mathematician, the next Einstein or the next Picasso to feel good about their efforts - we should encourage and praise where they are while also encouraging them positively to strive for better, in a supportive way.

I will present here the case of Deeana. Deeana is a young lady who had high hopes of doing a great job at school. She wanted to achieve high grades and she wanted to do well and get into a great University but there were always things coming into her way, distracting her, as she told me one day. For example, she had a very loud and boisterous family, making it hard for her to work, there were tenants in the adjacent area where they lived, causing so much noise Deeana couldn't sleep some nights, and she had a brother who would drink a lot and come home cursing, throwing her school papers in the garbage. Try studying after someone has ripped up your study notes. What was Deeana to do? She prayed. She prayed deeply and intensely for the Lord to help her through her problem and to take away all the distractions around her, all the challenges preventing her from doing all that she could. One by one, the distractions fell away: the other tenants moved out, causing for a much quieter living space, her parents learned that they were being inconsiderate and that they needed to lower their voices, and her brother spent time in rehab, taking care of his drinking problem. Deeana ended up graduating at the top of her class and to this day, as she is completing her Doctorate, she thanks God and relies on Him in every way and for all of her needs.

> Our family and our environment make a very big difference in who we end up being and so as parents and as children, we need to do our best to be our best and we also need to pray to God that He will help us after we have done all that we can to help ourselves.

What If I Didn't Come From the "Right" Family?

Many ask, *"Christine, what if I didn't come from the 'right' family, didn't have the right breaks growing up, didn't have any support?"* This can of course happen too and if that is you, not to worry, God has seen it all. He knows exactly what you've been through, how hard it was, how unsupportive and downright destructive factors in your life have been and here is the good news: **God has the final say on your success.** He will bring you that scholarship, He will bring you that job that will catapult you years ahead, He will make up for the lost childhood, He will be the dad or mom you never had. God will always be there to love you, to help you, to see you through everything you need. He will never abandon you, forsake you, leave you to fend for yourself, no matter what your family life or life has been like. No matter what sorts of injustices you have been through. He is on the throne, there, ready and willing and waiting to help you. All you have to do is ask through prayer.

Dr. Christine Topjian is a Toronto-based Award-Winning Author and enjoys helping people find their way, their voice and their relationship with the Lord. As one who grew up without much understanding of faith, she now enjoys helping people to discover all that is available in a loving relationship with Christ.

You can read more about her and find more of her titles at DrChristineTopjian.com.

She is also the Founder of free video-sharing website, YouBroadcaster.com.

www.ingramcontent.com/pod-product-compliance
Lightning Source LLC
Chambersburg PA
CBHW071855160426
13209CB00005B/1064